Cross Training

CROSS
TRAINING

R. G. "Nick" McNickle

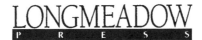

Photography by Maria Ferrari,
Ferrari Studio, NY, NY

DISCLAIMER

Before beginning this or any other exercise program, first
check with your physician.

Copyright © 1994 by R. G. McNickle

Published by Longmeadow Press, 201 High Ridge Road,
Stamford, CT 06904. All rights reserved. No part of this
book may be reproduced or utilized in any form or by
any means, electronic or mechanical, including photo-
copying, recording or by any information storage and
retrieval system, without permission in writing from the
Publisher.

Cover design by Kelvin P. Oder

Library of Congress Cataloging-in-Publication Data

McNickle, R. G.
    Cross training / R.G. "Nick" McNickle. — 1st ed.
        p. cm.
    ISBN: 0-681-41686-6
    1. Physical education and training. 2. Exercise.
3. Physical fitness. I. Title.
GV711.5.M38   1994
613.7'11—dc20   93-21650
                                                      CIP

Printed in United States of America

First Edition

0 9 8 7 6 5 4 3 2 1

TO DAD

Acknowledgments

W hen she was attending St. Joseph's College Mom
majored in Latin and for the last twenty-five years
of his life Dad was a copy editor in the New York Times
Sports Department. While Mom helped with "school and
sports" as she put it, neither she nor Dad ever insisted that
their boys concentrate on the English language above all
else. But the influence of one's parents runs deep. With the
completion of this book I now join brothers Mike and Chris
as the third son who writes for publication. I thank them,
and Mom, deeply for their strong support over all the years,
particularly the last two while I was writing.

The heroine behind this book is my wonderful wife
Litna. My greatest gratitude goes to Litna for the many
fourteen hour work days she put in caring for Daniel, Katie
and Rebecca so that I would have time to collect information and write about cross training. My thanks to Daniel

and Katie and Rebecca for their spirit and patience throughout the stages of the project. I promise I won't sign up to write another book—for a while.

Much of my time writing was spent at my mother-in-law's. Cloty, her mother Ita, and brother-in-law Tom helped me stay the course through their feedback, nourishment, and genuine interest in the book's progress.

When I was a physical education major at Herbert H. Lehman College in the Bronx several outstanding professors fostered my growth. I would like to thank especially Ted Hurwitz and Edwin Kramer for their help then and over the years. Exercise physiologist Joseph DiGennaro was instrumental in stimulating my desire to continue learning how the human body works, and advisor Harv Ebel guided me through the very rewarding process of writing a Master's Degree thesis.

At John Jay College it has been my good fortune to be surrounded by dedicated physical educators and coaches since 1976. Had it not been for Department Chairperson Susan Larkin's willingness to let our department undertake the New York City Female Firefighter Training Program in the summer of 1988, it is doubtful whether I ever would have been approached by Dorothy Regan of Longmeadow Press. So, for Sue's willingness to accept a daunting challenge, and for her long term support of many activities within the Cardiovascular Fitness Center, I am most grateful.

Fellow exercise physiologists and accomplished triathletes Mikki McNulty and John Conboy were generous with their advice as I wrestled with understanding and explaining a new approach to exercise. Diane Conboy also provided a sympathetic ear when I was revved up about completing another step in this project.

For the professional example they have set and for their friendship over many years I would like to thank John Jay College colleagues Bob Fox, Bob Fletcher, Jeff Risener, Tony Phillips, Lou DeMartino, Joe Schutz, Wallace Pina, and Dan Jesmur. More recently I have come to admire the commitment to teaching and promoting exercise demonstrated by Johanna Forman, Jane Katz, Dave Umeh, Shannon Whalen and Ulana Lysniak. Tizita Ayele, Teri Freaney, Zobeida Altagracia, and Tyrone Oree have been most helpful within our department as well.

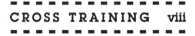

In the summer of 1989 Gail Stentiford of New York University was kind enough to give me the opportunity to begin teaching a wonderful adult exercise class called Exercise Prescription. More than a few of the ideas in this book were developed to help students in the Exercise Prescription class. NYU Professor of Sociology Caroline Persell is an accomplished author who has taken the class several times. Caroline empathized with the inevitable frustrations of a novice writer. Even as she did her Monark bike workout she offered excellent suggestions which helped keep me going.

Many friends took a sincere interest in the progress of Cross Training and I would like to thank them for their enthusiasm: Elven and Diane Riley, David and Leah Bekier, Pat and Mary Fava, and Nelson and Debbie Serrano.

I would like to express great appreciation to my editor, Pamel Liflander, for all of her work to make Cross Training a better book. Pam's gift for pushing gently but firmly helped me to meet several deadlines. She would be a talented personal trainer. Thanks too to copy editor Erin Clermont for her mammoth efforts.

I owe a particularly large debt of gratitude to photographer Maria Ferrari for contributing many hours to this endeavor. I thank Pedro Arroyo for doing the sketches and for being a model for the photographs. I would also like to acknowledge the members of John Jay College's Cardiovascular Fitness Center who were kind enough to volunteer their time to be models for the photographs: Darcy Aldrich, Venus Baerga, Paul Gjioni, Terence Holden, Ann Kuhn, Mike McInnis, Pat Mongiello, Ismael Morales, and Judy-Lynne Peters.

Finally, I would like to acknowledge my students at John Jay College and New York University, the faculty and staff members of the John Jay College Fitness Center, and the faculty and staff at John Jay College who are not yet exercising. You were all my audience as I wrote Cross Training. I imagined I was speaking directly to you with three goals: One, to help the inactive learn to enjoy exercise. Two, to guide active exercisers into a new exciting and rewarding approach to their workouts. And three, to explain to those already doing more than one activity how to cross train better.

Contents

History of
Cross Training

Cross training is adding another physical activity to your primary form of exercise. The two (or more) activities can be performed daily, weekly, or seasonally.

When NBA great Michael Jordan does his twenty-minute weight-lifting workout the morning of a game, he is performing daily cross training for the benefit of enhanced sports performance. Cross training is also effective on a weekly basis. For example, the recreational jogger can cross train by doing a twenty-minute workout on a stationary exercise cycle once a week. Or the same jogger can follow the instructions for cross training with swimming (Chapter 11) and build up to a twenty-minute swim once a week. In this way cross training provides a counterpoint to boredom. In addition, cross training reduces injuries, develops better overall physical fitness, offers new challenges, instills confidence, fosters friendships, strengthens personal relationships, and opens new time and location workout options.

Although the term *cross training* was not coined until the 1980s, athletes have been experiencing the cross-training challenge since the pentathlons of ancient Greece, which put athletes through a series of physical tests of strength, speed, and stamina. In the 1912 Olympic Games in Stockholm, the legendary Jim Thorpe won both the pentathlon and the decathlon. After his Olympic feats, Thorpe went on to play major league baseball and professional football; in 1950 the Associated Press voted him the greatest athlete of the half-century. Thorpe's broad scope of cross training was approached by Jim Brown, who excelled in basketball and lacrosse at Syracuse University and took tenth place in the 1954 Amateur Athletic Union National Decathlon Championship. He went on to a brilliant professional football career.

The record holder in the decathlon is sometimes called "the world's greatest athlete," which would make Dan O'Brien the top cross-training athlete of our time. But a strong case could be made on behalf of Mark Allen, master of three sports and current Ironman Triathlon champion. And let us not forget the recent achievements of football/baseball stars Bo Jackson and Deion Sanders.

"Babe" Didrikson Zaharias set cross-training records in the 1930s and 1940s when she earned national recognition in basketball, set world records in track and field (winning two Olympic gold medals), and captured every major women's golf championship. In 1950 the Associated Press voted Zaharias the top female athlete of the half-century; no female athlete since has matched the standard of cross training she achieved. Perhaps closest to Zaharias is Jackie Joyner-Kersee. After Kersee's 1992 Olympic gold medal performance in the heptathlon, former decathlon champion Bruce Jenner said that Joyner-Kersee had proved herself "the greatest multievent athlete ever, man or woman."

Cross Training opens the doors of this exciting sports regimen to everyone. Whether you are a novice or an expert at any one particular activity, read on and explore the possibilities cross training offers.

2

Benefits of Cross Training

B y its very nature, cross training brings balance to your exercise routine. Working muscle groups that you normally don't use permits those muscles that are well toned to take a break. When a runner cross trains by exchanging a run for a swim workout or a cyclist cross trains by exchanging a ride for a rowing workout, the athlete is lessening the risk of an overuse injury. Since overtraining accounts for a high percentage of exercise injuries, cross training represents a significant benefit by reducing trauma.

Injury Prevention

If you should injure one body part—your knee, for example—with cross training you may be able to continue exercising without performing the movement that hurts your knee. You will maintain your conditioning while you heal. Josh Tankel is a passionate cyclist who has averaged fifty to seventy miles per week on his racing bike, eight months per year since 1980. His knees, however, can no longer stand this volume of exercise. His best cross-training option is to swim or do some other water-based activity, such as hydroaerobics or water running while his knees get their much needed rest. Some cyclists with knee problems are able to do knee extension and knee flexion exercises on training machines to maintain leg strength during the healing process. These exercises work the upper leg muscles, but at a different angle than cycling, avoiding the aggravation associated with overtraining.

Physical Fitness Benefits

In addition to reducing injuries, the balance of cross training contributes strongly to all-round physical fitness. The runner whose upper body has been ignored for years can add swimming, rowing, or strength training as correct cross-training alternatives and will soon have a better overall muscular profile.

A well-organized cross-training exercise program will develop each of the five components of physical fitness: aerobic fitness, muscular strength, muscular endurance, flexibility, and body composition. Evaluate your current exercise routine against all five components. If your current routine is inadequate or incomplete in respect to any component of physical fitness, then you can add the appropriate cross-training activity that will lead to a better balanced exercise program.

Aerobic Fitness

Aerobic fitness (also referred to as cardiovascular fitness) is probably the most important component of physical fitness because of its relationship to high-quality health. A good cardiovascular system decreases your chance of heart disease, the leading cause of death in the United States.

Aerobic fitness is developed by engaging in an activity that takes your heart rate to your target zone for twenty minutes or more, three times per week at least. (Chapter 3 lists fifty sports and activities that provide aerobic fitness.)

Benefits of Aerobic Exercise

- Stronger, healthier heart
- Increases the amount of blood pumped per beat (stroke volume) at rest and during exercise
- Improves elasticity in blood vessel walls
- Increases maximum oxygen consumption
- Improves blood lipid profile
- Induces the "runner's high" from endorphins (other endurance activities performed at sufficient intensity may offer this sensation as well)
- Relieves stress, elevates mood
- Helps clear arteries of plaque (reduces atherosclerosis)
- Normalizes blood pressure
- Decreases resting heart rate
- Decreases percentage of body fat

Strength

Absolute strength is measured by the maximum force you can generate with one all-out effort; for example, the maximum number of pounds you can lift on one attempt. Developing a reasonable level of strength is important because it will lead to greater physical work capacity, less chance of certain types of injuries, less chance of lower back problems, better posture, and, in an emergency, make you better able to respond successfully.

Benefits of Strength Training

- Improves functional fitness
- Improves muscle tone
- Improves posture

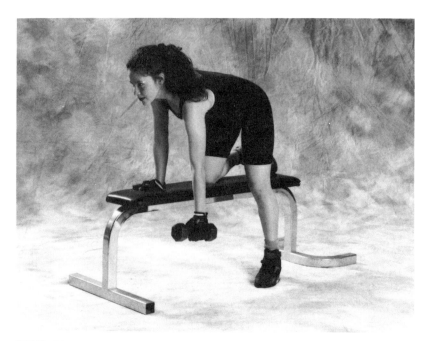

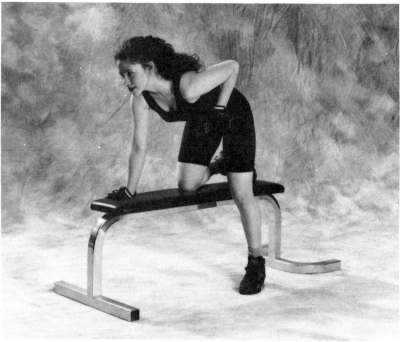

If you choose to add weight lifting to your weekly routine balanced physical fitness will be one of your cross training benefits.

- Improves blood circulation to bones, joints, and spinal disks
- Increases bone density, preventing osteoporosis
- Reduces risk of lower back problems

Muscular Endurance

Muscular endurance is a muscle's ability to contract and relax repeatedly. It is usually measured by the number of times (repetitions) you can perform a movement in a set time. Abdominal muscles are frequently utilized to assess muscular endurance via the one-minute sit-up test. Good muscular endurance can improve the static strength of your bones, ligaments, and tendons.

Flexibility

Flexibility is a measure of the range of motion at a joint or group of joints. Muscle length affects this range of motion, so the stretching capacity of your muscles plays an important role in flexibility. Relative to the other four components of physical fitness, flexibility is probably the least publicized. While good flexibility is essential to top performance in many sports, there is no one sport or activity that highlights flexibility the way the mile race focuses on cardiovascular fitness or Olympic weight lifting focuses on strength. National and world-class performers and athletes with good coaches are usually required to address flexibility each workout because the coach or trainer insists on it. The recreational athlete usually works without a coach, however, and unfortunately tends to undervalue the need for *flexibility training.* Developing and maintaining flexibility should be thought of in the same focused manner as aerobic training and strength training.

Cross training can help. The walker who adds two aerobic dance classes to the weekly routine simply for the additional range of motion in several joints will be automatically addressing the flexibility issue.

Benefits of Flexibility Training

- Improves functional fitness
- Improves sport performance
- Reduces risk of injury

Body Composition

Body composition is the fifth component of physical fitness and refers to the relative percentage of muscle, fat, bone, and other tissues that make up the human body. Some studies have estimated that as many as 50 percent of American adults are too fat. The good news is that all aerobic cross-training activities improve body composition by reducing the percentage of body fat. Strength-training and muscular-endurance workouts improve body composition by increasing the cross section (thickness) of the muscles and by enhancing muscle tone. If you combine aerobic cross-training, strength-training, and muscular-endurance workouts with a carefully planned diet, you will be able to improve your body composition.

Psychological Benefits of Cross Training

Cross training is psychologically stimulating because it provides variety in your exercise regime. It is an excellent method of training for serious athletes whose workouts have gone stale. A change of pace is refreshing and allows any athlete to be excited about working out again.

As you master your cross-training routine, in particular the new cross-training activity you have chosen, you will feel a sense of accomplishment and begin thinking about your next cross-training activity challenge.

New Friends and Relationships

As you try new activities you will meet other exercisers and make new friends. You will continue to work out with your primary activity training partners, but at the same time you will have the opportunity to develop new relationships

If you have been doing your workouts alone because your spouse or friend does not enjoy your primary activity, or it just isn't available at your current workout time, how about discussing a cross-training alternative that you would both enjoy and could do together?

New Time and Location Workout Options

With cross training, the tennis player can improve his cardiovascular fitness, muscular endurance, and flexibility without getting on the tennis court. Even when it's dark or raining, or all the courts are taken, the tennis player is still improving the physical conditioning aspect of his or her game.

If you select an aerobic cross-training option that can be done inside, on a piece of equipment you can afford (such as a stationary cycle ergometer, a rowing machine, a cross-country ski machine, a step-climbing machine, or a slide board, you greatly increase your time-of-day workout options.

If you can purchase a home version multiple-station strength-training machine, or even a pair of dumbbells, you will be able to do muscular development cross training at home, giving yourself additional time-of-day workout options.

The Physiology of Cross Training

The emphasis on engaging and developing underutilized muscle groups is the key way the physiology of cross training differs from the physiology of single-activity aerobic training. The improvement in overall physical fitness that cross training provides has already been discussed; adding activities that emphasize neglected areas of fitness should lead to balanced fitness. But what about the numerous athletes who claim cross training has contributed to new personal achievements in their primary sport? Frank Shorter (Olympic gold medalist, marathon), Mike Gratton (champion marathoner), Mark Nenow (10,000-meter

American record holder), Jennifer Hinshaw (nationally ranked swimmer), Debbie Henrickson (national age-group cycling sport champion), and Joy Hansen (professional triathlete), have each gone on record regarding physiological changes and improvements as a result of cross training. Do the successes of these very talented athletes mean that cross training should be thought of as a proven breakthrough in the science of physical training?

Even with the considerable evidence available, the answer to this question at this time has to be no. While the results the athletes describe are real, the cross-training programs were not conducted in a systematic manner. Controlled studies are needed to examine the precise effects of cross training, but it is difficult for physiologists to find athletes who will redesign their workout program for the sake of science.

For now, cross training represents a method of training that athletes of all levels can integrate into their exercise programs and evaluate. However, since properly performed aerobic cross training follows the well-established principles of intensity, frequency, duration, and progression, certain physiological training effects can be expected (after a minimum of twelve weeks of exercise). Keep in mind that the more oxygen the body can provide to your muscles the greater your capacity for muscular work. These physiological changes account for several of the benefits of aerobic exercise listed earlier and occur in four areas:

1. At the tissue level (biochemical)
• Increased myoglobin content

One muscle tissue adaptation is an increase in a molecule complex found in the blood called myoglobin, which is responsible for the muscle's ability to store oxygen. The myoglobin binds with oxygen and aids the delivery of oxygen from the cell membrane to the mitochondria, organisms that provide the principal source of cellular energy "energy factories."

• Increased oxidation of carbohydrates (glycogen)

Oxidation is any process in which the oxygen content of a compound is increased. The increased oxidation of carbohydrates means more oxygen is available to the working muscles. In other words, the capacity of the muscle to generate energy aerobically is improved. Also, the muscle's ability to store carbohydrates is increased.

- **Increased oxidation of fat**

Fat serves as a major source of fuel for skeletal muscle during endurance exercises. Therefore, an increased capacity to oxidize (make use of) fat is an advantage in increasing the performance of such activities.

2. **Within the circulatory and respiratory systems**
   - **Changes in the heart: increased stroke volume and decreased resting heart rate**

Stroke volume is the amount of blood ejected by the left ventricle per beat. Aerobic training increases stroke volume at rest and during exercise. The increased stroke volume at rest means the heart does not need to pump as often for any fixed period of time when compared with an untrained heart. Over the course of a lifetime this physiological change reduces the wear on the heart. The increased stroke volume during exercise provides greater aerobic work capacity.

   - **Increased blood volume**

Your blood carries oxygen throughout your body. Having a greater volume of blood available to the working muscles increases their work capacity.

   - **Increased capillary density**

Capillaries are tiny blood vessels that join the end of an artery to the beginning of a vein. Having more capillaries per muscle fiber enhances the supply of oxygen to the muscle and the removal of waste products from the muscle.

3. **In the blood chemistry lowers blood cholesterol and triglyceride levels**

Cholesterol is a fat soluble substance widely distributed in the body that has been associated with higher risk of heart disease when levels exceed 200 milligrams/deciliter. Triglycerides are blood fat compounds also found in the blood and are considered important in the diagnosis and treatment of diabetes, hypertension, and heart disease. The total amount of triglyceride in the blood is normally less than 300 milligrams/deciliter.

Regular aerobic exercise programs cause decreases in both blood cholesterol and triglyceride levels.

4. In the blood pressure : may reduce high blood pressure

Blood pressure is the force exerted by the blood against the walls of the arteries. It is measured in millimeters of mercury (mm/Hg). A normal blood pressure for an adult might be *120/80 mm Hg*. The 120 refers to the systolic blood pressure, which is measured when the heart is contracting (the systole phase). The 80 refers to the diastolic blood pressure, which is measured between contractions of the heart when the blood is entering the relaxed chambers (the diastole phase). Diastolic blood pressure may vary with age, body weight, emotional state, and time of day.

High blood pressure for adults is considered to begin at 140/90 mm Hg (this level is frequently referred to as borderline hypertension). Individuals with hypertension show significant reductions in resting systolic and diastolic blood pressure after adding regular aerobic exercise to their lifestyles.

3

The Principles of Exercise and Cross Training

The combination of activities that will make cross training work for you should include at least one activity that can be performed aerobically.

Aerobic exercise is continuous in nature and is performed at an intensity at which the oxygen needs of the working muscles are being met throughout the workout. When performed at a moderate intensity, walking, jogging, cycling, swimming, aerobic dance, in-line skating, and step classes are examples of aerobic exercise activities.

Selection of the actual aerobic sport or activity that can be performed aerobically is the first principle of cross training. There are four primary principles for aerobic activity: intensity, frequency, duration, and progression.

Intensity of Training:
How Hard Are You Working?

The intensity of your exercise session may be measured by your heart-rate response to exercise or by your rating of perceived exertion.

Measuring your heart rate response involves taking your pulse right after you stop exercising and counting the number of beats you feel in fifteen seconds. Since the heart is a muscle, it can be strengthened by aerobic exercise performed at a certain minimum intensity. Exercise physiologists' understanding of the effect on the heart of different exercise intensity levels led to the development of a concept known as the *target heart rate zone.*

During your aerobic training you will raise your heart rate from a typical resting rate of 70 beats per minute to your target heart rate. Your target heart rate is based on your age and may be calculated easily with the following formula:

$$\frac{220 - \text{Your age}}{} = \text{Maximum heart rate (predicted)}$$

To find out your exact maximum heart rate you would need to take a special exercise test with an electrocardiogram machine. This test is also known as a "stress test."

To calculate the lower end of your target heart rate zone multiply your maximum heart rate by .7.

To calculate the upper end of your target heart zone multiply your maximum heart rate by .85.

Calculations for a 40-Year-Old Exerciser:

```
 220
 −40 (age)
 180 = Maximum heart rate (predicted)

 180
x  .7 (70% of maximum heart rate)
 126 = Lower end of target heart rate zone

 180
x .85 (85% of maximum heart rate)
 153 = Upper end of target heart rate zone
```

The target heart rate zone for our forty-year-old exerciser doing aerobic cross training is 126 to 153.

You can find your pulse with the two fingers of your writing hand at your radial artery, on the inside of your opposite wrist. Or you can find your pulse at your carotid artery on the side of your neck (place your fingers gently on your neck). After you have found your pulse, count the number of beats you feel for fifteen seconds and multiply that number by four. This simple calculation tells you your exercise heart rate. For your first two areobic cross-training workouts you should calculate your exercise heart rate after five minutes of your workout, after ten minutes, and after twenty minutes. If your exercise heart rate is below the lower end of your target heart rate, you may want to try to work a little harder, if you feel up to it. If your target heart rate is above the upper end of your target heart rate zone, you should reduce the intensity of your efforts and thus lower your exercise heart rate.

Rating of Perceived Exertion (RPE)

Rating of Perceived Exertion is a method for evaluating how hard *you feel* you are working. As most people find it easy to perceive accurately the physical costs of different workloads, you may want to make use of the Brog Perceived Exertion Scale. It can be fun to make your own subjective evaluation of how hard you exercise. The RPE helps put you in touch with your body; it helps you learn to listen to your body.

After you have mastered taking your pulse and working within your target heart rate zone, you will be ready to use the RPE scale. Just do your aerobic activity at a steady pace and make a judgment as to how hard you *feel* you are working.

Borg's Rating of Perceived Exertion Scale

6
7   Extremely light
8
9   Very light
10
11   Light
12
13   Somewhat hard
14
15   Hard (heavy)
16
17   Very hard
18
19   Extremely hard
20

(From Borg GA: Med Sci Sports Exerc 14:377-387, 1982. © The American College of Sports Medicine.)

If you rate your perceived exertion somewhere between 11 and 16, your exercise heart rate is probably equal to your RPE x 10 plus 20 to 30 beats per minute. Rating perceived exertion will be useful to you because it increases your awareness of how workouts can vary in intensity. There will be days when you begin to exercise and you sense right away you are not feeling up to a vigorous workout (RPE = 14 or more). It's O.K. to lower your intensity and do an easy workout (RPE = 8 to 11).

Frequency

Considerable research has demonstrated that three aerobic exercise sessions per week are needed to gain the cardiorespiratory benefits of aerobic exercise. Therefore, whether doing traditional aerobic training (the same activity three times per week) or cross training (adding or substituting different activities), three aerobic workouts should be your minimum weekly goal.

Duration

Again, the research done examining the dose-response phenomena of exercise provides us with needed guidelines. It has been demonstrated that twenty minutes of continuous exercise (performed three times per week) provides cardiorespiratory benefits. Thus, the aerobic portion of your workout should last for twenty minutes. When you add a warm-up of about 5 to 10 minutes; muscular development 10 to 15 minutes; and a cooldown of 5 to 10 minutes, the typical cross-training workout will take approximately 45 minutes.

Progression

Your rate of progression will depend on your aerobic capacity, your health status, your age, your needs, and your goals. Aerobic cross training has three stages of progression: the beginning stage, the improvement stage, and maintenance.

Beginning Stage

The beginning stage of your workouts will be distinguished by a relatively low level of intensity and slight muscle soreness (after a few weeks you will wake up without soreness as the muscles become accustomed to the movements of exercise). Relatively low intensity means that it is fine for you to stay toward the lower end of your target heart rate zone and at about 11 or 12 on the Rating of

Perceived Exertion scale. You risk injury if you go too hard too soon. Since you are not going to be in shape after one week of exercise anyway, why not ease into your training program and keep muscle soreness to a minimum?

This beginning conditioning stage will usually last from four to six weeks. During this stage, you should check your pulse after five minutes and again after ten minutes during the aerobic phase of each workout. If your pulse is at the lower end of your target heart rate zone, and you feel OK, you are probably on the right track. If your pulse is near the upper end of your target heart rate zone, or if you are experiencing too much discomfort to enjoy the workout, you should reduce your effort slightly.

During the beginning conditioning stage it is fine to modify your workout and do only ten or fifteen minutes of aerobic exercise. Divide your aerobic workout into five-minute segments if you wish. As you feel able increase to four five-minute segments, then modify those to two ten-minute segments, and then progress to twenty continuous minutes.

Completing twenty minutes of continuous aerobic exercise at target heart rate intensity could be your first goal. After you achieve a goal you should congratulate yourself, give yourself a reward if you wish, and begin thinking about setting a new goal.

The ability to perform twenty minutes of continuous aerobic exercise can be used as a milepost to signify the end of the beginning conditioning stage.

Improvement Stage

The improvement conditioning stage occurs immediately after the completion of the beginning stage and is marked by rapid progesss in your primary activity. As you find yourself handling the same intensity of exercise more easily, you will see that your heart rate for that level of exercise will be lower. To stimulate your heart rate so that it will be in your target zone, you will have to increase the intensity of your primary activity; these increases may be needed every few weeks for up to four months.

Maintenance

After around six months of aerobic cross training you will probably be physically ready to begin the maintenance

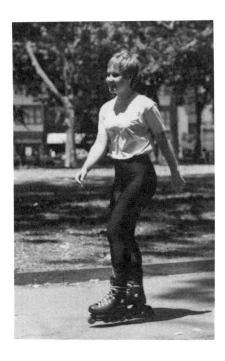

In-line skating is just one of your many aerobic cross training options.

conditioning stage. If you decide at this point that you are not interested in additional increases in your intensity level, you may continue your workout routine and maintain aerobic fitness. By this time you may have made a decision regarding your favorite primary activity and will settle into a consistent workout schedule that calls for only one or two days of cross training per week. Many exercisers develop an excellent, enjoyable maintenance conditioning program.

There is another type of conditioning program you may be interested in at this point—long-term improvement conditioning. Reaching your full physical potential can take years of training. If this comes to be one of your challenges, try setting achievable goals that extend your abilities. As you reach the goal, take pride in your success, take a little time off if you wish, and set your next goal. When do you stop? It's up to you. Some exercisers would rather switch activities than go into a standard maintenance program.

Fifty Aerobic Fitness Activities

1. Aerobic Dance
2. Backpacking
3. Badminton
4. Basketball
5. Boxing
6. Canoeing
7. Cross-Country Skiing (machine)
8. Cross-Country Skiing (outdoors)
9. Cycling (outdoors)
10. Cycling (stationary bike)
11. Duathlon (run, bike, run)
12. Fencing
13. Field Hockey
14. Golf (walk and carry bag)
15. Handball
16. Hiking
17. Horseback Riding (trot or gallop)
18. Hydroaerobics
19. Ice Skating
20. In-line Skating
21. Judo
22. Karate (competition)
23. Kayaking
24. Lacrosse
25. Mountain Climbing
26. Paddleball
27. Racquetball
28. Rope Jumping
29. Rowing (machine)
30. Rowing (outdoors)
31. Rugby
32. Running
33. Scuba Diving
34. Slide Boarding (indoors)
35. Snowboarding
36. Snowshoeing
37. Soccer
38. Social Dancing
39. Squash
40. Stair Climbing
41. Step Class
42. Step Climbing (machine)
43. Swimming
44. Tennis
45. Treadmill Running
46. Triathlon
47. Versa Climber (machine)
48. Volleyball
49. Walking
50. Water Running

Anaerobic Exercise

Many sports do not have continuous action, but the rest periods are so short that your aerobic energy system is in operation throughout the game. Basketball and handball are good examples of such sports.

If the intensity of play increases enough you will be working so hard that the oxygen supply to your muscles will not be sufficient to maintain the aerobic state. At that point you will be exercising anaerobically. This is a normal response to vigorous physical exertion. An anaerobic process is one that does not require the utilization of oxygen. You will know when you are exercising anaerobically because you will start to breathe very deeply and quickly. You are trying to bring in enough oxygen so that your muscles can work aerobically but it doesn't happen. Your body will only allow you to work anaerobically for a few minutes. This is because during anaerobic exercise you generate energy at a rate greater than you are entitled to according to your oxygen intake. There is a limit to the amount of oxygen debt you can incur, and the lactic acid produced during anaerobic exercise causes pain in the muscles.

Interval Training

Even though anaerobic exercise is more strenuous than aerobic exercise many athletes seeking to maximize speed performance incorporate it into their workouts through interval training. Interval training is based on the concept that the correct spacing of work and rest periods enables you to accomplish a tremendous amount of exercise over a considerable period of time with minimal fatigue. The rest-to-work intervals can be as little as ten seconds or as long as several minutes. The training prescription can vary in terms of intensity and duration of the exercise interval, the time allowed for the recovery period, and the number of repetitions.

During the intervals a rather severe workload can be imposed on the muscles and oxygen transport system. But before the lactic acid has accumulated to the point where it would prevent further exercise, you begin a recovery period. Your next work interval begins after this brief recovery.

Interval training is considered fundamental to improving speed performance. You will find athletes of all levels doing interval training to become faster. Sprint swimmers, for example, do intervals at a distance one-quarter or half as long as their event. A 100-yard free-styler will swim numerous intervals of 25 and 50 yards at 95 to 100 percent effort interspersed with "rest" periods of 15 seconds or less. A triathlete training for a one-mile swim would do 100 and 200 yard intervals.

Specificity of Training

Your metabolism is a series of vital processes in which the energy and nutrients from foods are utilized by your body. Specificity of training refers to adaptations in your metabolic and physiologic systems that reflect the type of training you have done. An activity that develops primarily one area of fitness should not be expected, by itself, to contribute much to the other four components of physical fitness. You can do scores of sit-ups to strengthen your stomach muscles without improving your capacity for aerobic exercise.

This concept of specificity is important, too, for athletes who wish to reach their physical potential in any given sport. For example, if a handball player wishes to be a more accomplished competitor, he or she must play a lot of handball. Cross training by doing upper body muscular development exercises and sprint repeats will provide the handball player with many of the fitness demands of handball, but these cross-training activities will not improve the shot-making skills or the reflexes needed for success. To develop the skill aspect of any hand-eye or leg-eye sport, you must practice the sport. To develop the exact physical demands of any competitive event, you must perform those movements in training. To run faster, jump higher, or swim farther, you must do many workouts running fast, jumping high, and swimming far.

Cross training is valuable when you do it *before* you reach the point where your volume of training is going to cause an injury from overuse. How do you know when you are approaching this level of training? It is not easy to say. The athletes with the best records of long, relatively injury-free competitive careers (the champion hurdler Edwin Moses comes to mind), appear to be those who learn, early on, to listen to their bodies carefully. When a part of the body does not *feel* right, these athletes are able to sense it, and they are smart enough to make adjustments in their training schedule that allow healing to take place. Naturally, consultation with a sports medicine expert is a good idea if you feel some type of pain or have any physical problem that persists.

Developing better flexibility and greater strength can also contribute to a healthy exercise career. The relationship of cross training with each of these physical fitness components is the subject of the next two chapters.

4

Cross Training and Flexibility

Flexibility is the ability to move muscles and joints through their full range of motion. *Stretching* is the word often used to describe the various movements and maneuvers performed to enhance flexibility. Quality stretching should be part of your exercise program. You may think of it as "flexibility training" if you prefer a somewhat more sophisticated term, but the process is the same.

Your primary activity provides you with some flexibility benefits you would not have if you were completely sedentary. Brisk walking and jogging stretch muscles, tendons, and ligaments in your legs and shoulders. If you cross train with an activity that does not duplicate the movements of walking/jogging, you are adding more stretching to your fitness profile—and this is good for you. (From a flexibility-benefit perspective, backpacking, for example, is quite similar to walking/jogging and would not add much to your flexibility rating. Bowling with good form, playing a racquet sport, rock climbing, or taking a step class would all take your body through a whole serious of stretches different from walking/jogging, thereby enhancing your overall flexibility.)

In Chapter 6 you will be assessing your flexibility. If you find that even with your cross-training workouts you still feel the need to address a given muscle group you have a few options. You can add a third activity that provides the missing flexibility training, or you can select the appropriate stretch from the twelve described in this chapter.

There are benefits from better flexibility. By achieving a higher level of flexibility you are probably reducing your risk of injury during exercise, or even during daily living. Better flexibility improves what can be called "functional fitness." When you have to move a piece of furniture, change a tire, put a baby in a car seat, attend to your garden, or perform some other task included in everyday living, you will be able to do it more easily, without getting hurt.

Better flexibility may also lead to improved performance in your sport. Range of motion is critical to many movements in competitive sport. For example, a pitcher needs to be able to throw hard without getting hurt. He or she must be able to rotate the throwing arm backward at the shoulder joint. The better the rotational flexibility at the shoulder the greater speed the arm can generate. This speed is then transmitted to the ball. Think about your sport and you will undoubtedly be able to identify your flexibility needs.

You can achieve more flexibility through cross training with the proper mix of two or more activities—even if you spend very little time in a stretching session.

Here is what John Jerome says in his wonderful treatise on stretching, Staying Supple: The Bountiful Pleasures of Stretching (Bantam Books, 1987):

> At its most effective and most pleasurable, stretching is a meditative interlude, a productive place to put the mind for a while. The teaching of meditation isn't the purpose here, but the result sought by most meditative disciplines—the unkinking of the psyche, so to

speak—is not that different from that of a good stretch. Stretching works on the physical instead of the mental plane, but therefore works a lot more concretely than mental practices can ever be. The sensation of stretching—the signal from the tissues—can be a powerful aid to mental focus, drawing your attention back, with every increase in tension, to the site and process. And as meditation also demonstrates, paying that kind of attention is the route to the deepest (most pleasurable) level of result.

The matter of which stretches you should do could be debated. There are books that describe as many as three hundred different stretches (Michael Alter's excellent *Sport Stretch*, Leisure Press, 1990, has pictures and descriptions of 311 stretches and recommends specific stretches by sport).

The twelve stretches presented here have been carefully selected and address each of the major muscle groups. They are presented in a top-down sequence, which is biomechanically sound and easy to remember, but you can change the order as long as you go slowly. By no means are these stretches necessarily the twelve best stretches for everyone. Try them out and see which ones you like best. As you learn more about stretching you may find other stretches that feel good and add them to your stretching routine.

You will enjoy your stretching more if you remember these simple guidelines:

- Avoid stretching on a full stomach (empty your bladder and bowels if need be).
- Wear loose and comfortable clothing.
- Don't wear jewelry.
- Move slowly into each stretch.
- Breathe normally and exhale deeper as you move farther into the stretch.
- Hold each stretch for 20 to 30 seconds (opinions vary on the ideal time; listen to your own body and decide for yourself).

Stretching should feel good. Always. Period. If anything hurts, don't do it.

Shoulder

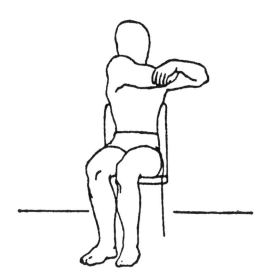

Perform sitting or standing.

- **R**aise one arm to shoulder height
- **F**lex your arm across to the opposite shoulder
- **G**rasp your raised elbow with the opposite hand
- **G**ently pull your elbow towards your body
- **H**old and relax

Triceps

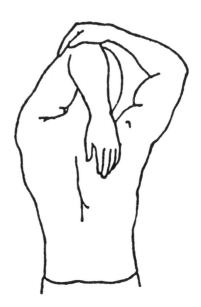

Perform sitting or standing.

- **F**lex one arm, raise it overhead next to your ear and let your hand rest on your shoulder blade.

- **G**rasp your elbow with the opposite hand and gently pull your elbow behind your head.

- **H**old and relax.

Chest

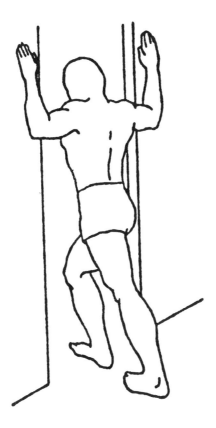

- **S**tand facing a corner or open doorway.
- **R**aise your arms to form a T.
- **L**ean forward with your entire body.
- **H**old and relax.

Upper Back

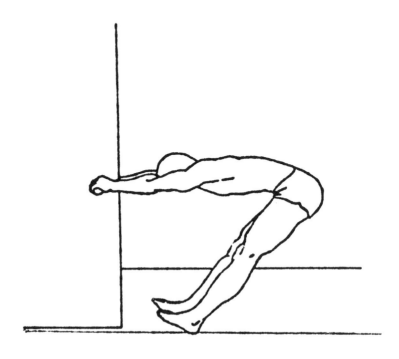

- **S**tand approximately 12 to 18 inches from an open door.
- **G**rasp the door handles with both hands.
- **K**eeping your feet flat on the ground and your knees bent, shift your hips backward and lower yourself until your arms are parallel to the ground.
- **H**old and relax.

Lateral Trunk

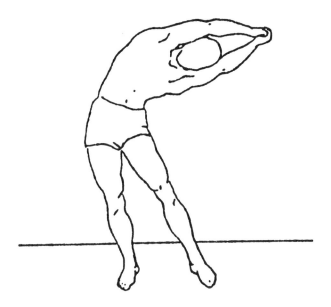

- **S**tand with feet slightly apart and hands touching overhead.
- **D**rop one ear toward your shoulder and slowly lower your arms sideways.
- **H**old and relax.

Lower Back

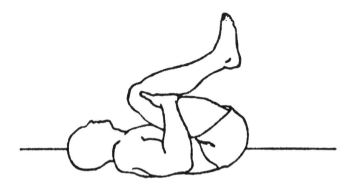

- **L**ie flat on your back with your hands at your sides and your legs extended.

- **B**end your knees and bring them up toward your chest.

- **G**rasp behind your thighs.

- **G**ently pull your knees in toward your chest. Your hips should roll up off the floor.

- **H**old and relax.

- **T**o complete the stretch, extend your legs slowly, one at a time.

Lower Back,
Gluteus Maximus, Hips

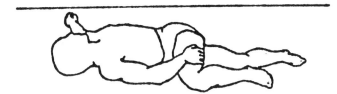

- **L**ie flat on your back with your legs extended.

- **F**lex one knee and raise it to your chest.

- **G**rasp your knee or thigh with one hand.

- **P**ull your knee across your body to the floor while keeping your elbows, head, and shoulders flat on the floor.

- **H**old and relax.

Lower Back and Hamstrings

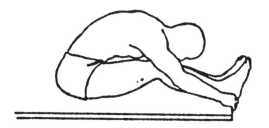

- **S**it down with knees slightly flexed.
- **S**lowly reach forward.
- **H**old and relax.

Hamstrings

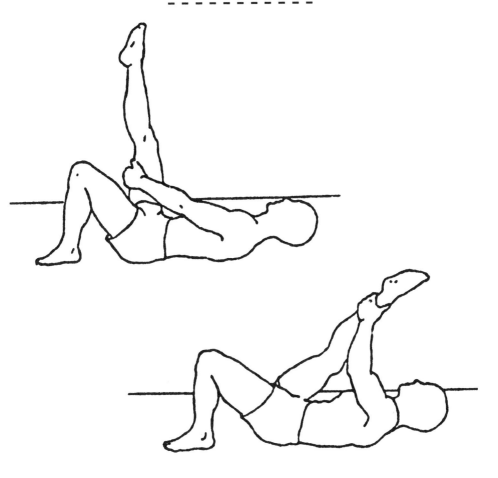

- **L**ie on your back, legs flexed and heels close to buttocks.
- **S**lowly extend one leg upward.
- **G**rasp underneath your leg.
- **G**ently pull the leg toward your face.
- **F**or a more thorough stretch, slowly straighten your leg.
- **H**old and relax.

Groin

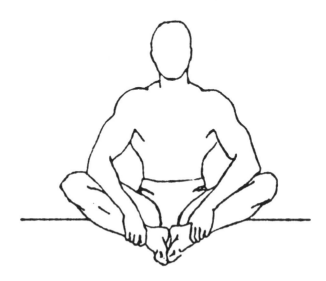

- **F**rom a sitting position, flex your knees and bring the soles of your feet together as you pull them toward your body.
- **P**lace your elbows on the inside portion of both upper legs.
- **S**lowly push your legs to the floor.
- **H**old and relax.

Quadriceps

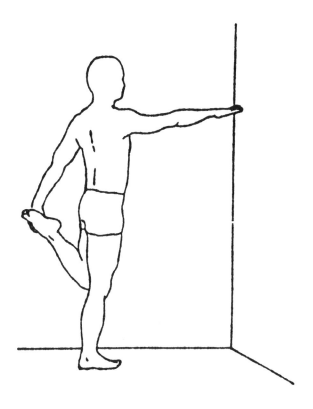

- **S**tand and place one hand against an object for balance.

- **B**end one knee and bring the foot up behind you.

- **K**eep the supporting leg slightly flexed.

- **R**each down and grasp your raised foot with one hand, then gently pull your heel toward your buttocks.

- **H**old and relax.

Calf

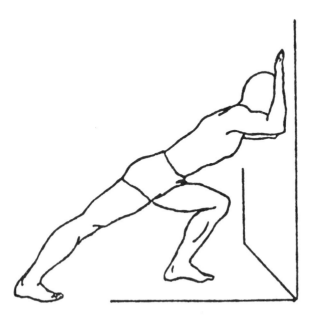

- **S**tand three to four feet from a wall.
- **S**tep forward with one leg (the knee will bend naturally) and keep the opposite leg straight.
- **L**ean against the wall maintaining the straight line of your head, neck, spine, and back leg.
- **K**eep your back foot flat.
- **F**lex your forward knee toward the floor.
- **H**old and relax.

5

Cross Training
for Strength

If you are doing any form of aerobic exercise on a regular basis and you add strength training, you are now cross training. As you head into your strength-training routine, it's helpful to have a positive mental attitude toward it. As with your primary aerobic activity and your stretching sessions, you should *enjoy* strength training. Take pride in every repetition. Enjoy the feeling of fatigue, or, if you want to work harder, exult in the soreness, knowing in your heart and your pectoralis major that you have worked hard. You are caring for your body by keeping it strong. Your muscles are meant to move, your figure is meant to flex, and if muscles had emotions they could express, after each workout they would say "Thanks, we needed that."

You have over six hundred muscles in your body; the classic medical text *Gray's Anatomy* devotes 160 pages

Major Muscles of Body *(Anterior)*

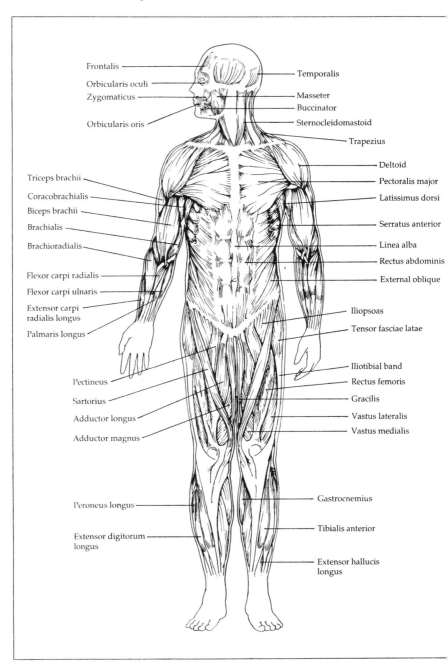

Frontalis
Orbicularis oculi
Zygomaticus
Orbicularis oris

Temporalis
Masseter
Buccinator
Sternocleidomastoid
Trapezius

Triceps brachii
Coracobrachialis
Biceps brachii
Brachialis
Brachioradialis
Flexor carpi radialis
Flexor carpi ulnaris
Extensor carpi radialis longus
Palmaris longus

Deltoid
Pectoralis major
Latissimus dorsi
Serratus anterior
Linea alba
Rectus abdominis
External oblique
Iliopsoas
Tensor fasciae latae

Pectineus
Sartorius
Adductor longus
Adductor magnus

Iliotibial band
Rectus femoris
Gracilis
Vastus lateralis
Vastus medialis

Peroneus longus
Extensor digitorum longus

Gastrocnemius
Tibialis anterior
Extensor hallucis longus

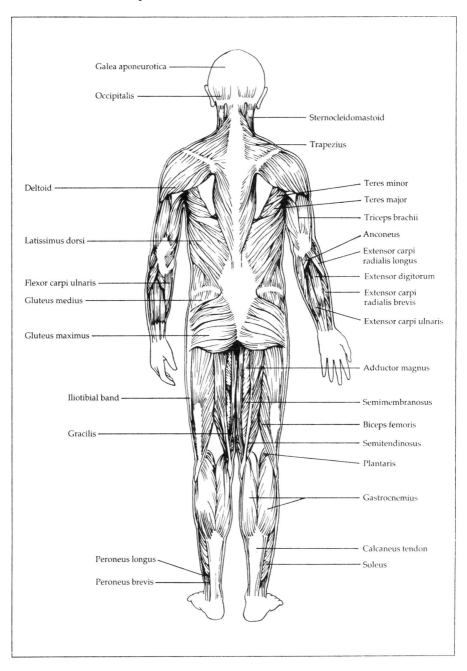

discussing them in detail. You may be pleased to know that to cross train for strength you need not know all the muscles of your body, but you do need to use them on a regular basis. The saying "Use it or lose it" applies to muscles in the strongest way. You will naturally come to know the major muscle groups as you train.

How do you go about developing a training plan to use six hundred muscles? You don't, actually. Two of the three types of muscles function involuntarily. Cardiac muscle (found only in the heart) and smooth muscle work for you without any conscious voluntary effort. Smooth muscle lines your hollow internal structures, such as blood vessels and the digestive tract. This chapter tells you about the importance of twelve major skeletal muscle groups. It is skeletal muscle that holds us together and allows us to move.

When you test your strength (see chapter 6) you will learn what it feels like to exert yourself in an all-out one-repetition maximum effort. This information is useful in setting up your strength-training workout. If for some reason you should not do one-rep max-strength testing, reading this chapter will show you how to organize an excellent strength-training workout without that information.

For example, if your primary sport or activity is listed in the index, you can look up how it is rated for upper and lower body strength on the Potential Physical Fitness Benefits chart. (see page 286) If your primary activity is using a step machine three times a week, you will see on the Fitness Benefits chart that your step machine workout does not provide upper body strength. Once you think about the movements of an activity you will usually be able to tell which muscles are involved. Then you can address the underutilized muscle groups in your strength-training workout. The resulting balanced physical fitness you will achieve will be worth the effort for a number of reasons.

In everyday living we are seldom called upon to perform an all-out muscular effort, but we do use our muscles for numerous activities, responsibilities, and chores. It is the ability to perform these everyday activities easily and safely—functional fitness, if you will—that represents the best reason to cross train for strength.

Greater Strength → Improved Functional Fitness → Better Ability:

- Play with and care for children, grandchildren, nieces and nephews
- Carry groceries
- Change a flat tire
- Paint a room
- Clean a house
- Tile a bathroom
- Mow a lawn
- Plant a garden
- Rake the leaves
- Wash and wax the car
- Lift a piece of furniture
- Move a heavy object (work related)
- Apprehend a bad guy (law enforcement)
- Fight a fire

On the importance of strength as it relates to leisure and occupational tasks, the American College of Sports Medicine states:

> The maintenance of enhancement of muscle strength and muscular endurance enables the individual to perform such tasks with less physiological stress. Maintenance of adequate strength becomes an increasingly important issue with advancing age, which is associated with a loss of lean weight.

Lean weight refers to your body weight not including fat tissue. For purposes of functional fitness, bone density and muscle mass are paramount. Weight-bearing activities help keep bones strong and less susceptible to osteoporosis (reduced bone density). Weaker bones break and fracture more easily. And if you have less muscle mass, you have less strength.

For years doctors took it for granted that with aging came an inevitable decline in muscular capabilities. But if you cross train for strength you can stay strong, active, and healthy for your entire adult life. There is compelling evidence that the predominant reason for decline in physical performance by older people has been their reduction of activity. Just a few years ago Tufts University researchers put subjects ages 86 to 96 on a weight-training program designed to strengthen their legs. After only two months the participants had doubled, tripled, and quadrupled their leg strength.

Furthermore, about 80 percent of all lower back problems are caused by muscular weakness, so cross training for abdominal strength makes sense for adult exercisers of all ages.

Until recently, American society generally discouraged older people from doing anything vigorous. In an effort to show appreciation for our parents and grandparents, we unknowingly contributed to their physical decline. "Let me get that for you, Mom." "Don't walk with those packages, Grandpa. I'll pick you up and drive you." Fortunately, we are beginning to see some signs that people whose age was considered old fifteen years ago can still participate. Future Hall of Fame baseball pitcher Nolan Ryan of the Texas Rangers is in his mid-forties and can still strike out opponents half his age. Actor Jack Palance got a big laugh for doing one-armed pushups at the 1992 Academy Award, but some older men may have been thinking, If he can stay in shape, why can't I? As a nation, we need to continue to press ourselves hard to sustain this new outlook on aging and physical activity.

If you have parents and grandparents who have gradually eased into a minimum exertion lifestyle, you should pick up the challenge of encouraging your loved ones to stay active. Should Grandma begin using the manual lawn mower to trim half an acre of backyard grass? Probably not. But there are many less strenuous activities she could be doing that would be wonderful for her. Is Grandpa going to begin lifting barbells? Maybe. As mentioned above, people his age have had success with strength training. But you should at least encourage him to lift what he feels he can.

If you are recognizing yourself as a person who has drifted away from muscle-engaging activities, take this opportunity to reexamine your daily routine with respect to lifting, pushing, and pulling. Are there chores you could do for yourself that would let you get a few muscles moving? Are you strong minded enough to begin cross training for strength? Will you have an answer ready when you tell your non-exercising friends and family what you are doing and they look at you quizzically? "I feel better when I do my strength-training workouts" you will tell them (and you will). Ask a friend, "Why don't you come with me?" One day someone will and you will have done that person a great favor—besides getting a new workout partner for yourself.

You can tell the skeptics about Frank Spellman from Florida. In 1942, age twenty, Frank won the Junior National Championship for Olympic weight lifting. He competed in the middleweight division and weighed 165 pounds. At age seventy, Frank still weighs 165 pounds. He can squat 400 pounds five times and bench press 200 pounds ten times. Do you need to be able to lift this much weight to have functional fitness? No, but as a result of his strength training, Frank Spellman not only has excellent functional fitness for his everyday activities, he looks better, he feels better, and he is healthier.

What other group of people in the United States has been steered away from strength training? With only a few exceptions, such as swimming and ballet for school-age girls, women of all ages have been discouraged from most forms of exercise. In the 1960s, jogging and aerobic dance came on the scene and became socially correct for adult women, but strength training was taboo.

Now that we know that women can cross train for strength without fear of developing bulging biceps they should definitely do so. Ladies, you have less testosterone than men, and it is this hormone that plays a major role in increasing muscle size. You will achieve better muscle tone and functional fitness because your muscles will be stronger and firmer. Increasing the amount of muscle tissue on your body is good for weight control, too, because every pound of muscle you have requires 75 calories a day to keep it supplied with blood for nutrition and oxygen, whereas each pound of fat requires only 2 calories a day to keep it alive.

What is important to realize is that adults of all ages can and should maintain reasonable strength in their major muscle groups throughout life.

To train your muscles for greater strength you need to perform some form of exercise where muscles must offer resistance. The resistance can be provided by weights, machines, straps, bands, tubing, or a partner. The muscles, tendons, ligaments, and bones you use will gradually adapt to the resistance. You then gradually increase the resistance until you reach a level of strength and tone with which you are satisfied.

There are four ways you can cross train for strength:

1. Free weight
2. Machines
3. Straps, bands, tubing
4. Manual resistance provided by a partner

Free weight refers to using plates, barbells, and dumbbells of varying weight and combinations. Machines have weight stacks and you place a pin (or key) to set the amount of weight you want to lift. These two methods of strength training allow you to measure progress easily and precisely.

The principles of strength training apply to all four training methods.

• Specificity: "You get what you pay for"—the muscle groups you train are the muscle groups that get stronger, as long as you are following the principles of strength training described in this chapter. (Curiously, there have been studies showing the muscle tone of an immobilized limb to be positively affected by strength training with the opposite limb. Doctors have referred to this phenomenon as cross-lateral transfer but are not yet completely sure why or how it happens.)

• Intensity: You must exercise the muscle against a resistance sufficient to fatigue the muscle. If you want to develop your strength to its full potential you will need to exercise the muscle (or muscle group) to exhaustion. One formula for determining your initial intensity level is based on calculating 60 percent of your one-repetition maximum lift.

• Progression: This is also known as the progressive overload principle. Exercising your muscles at the appropriate intensity will stimulate cellular changes in those muscles as they adapt to the stress caused by a given resistance. If you were to continue exercising your muscles at the original intensity after they had adapted to the resistance, you would find it extremely difficult to gain additional strength. Progression means that as the muscles adapt, you set a new intensity or workload for them to resist. Progression is accomplished most often by lifting greater weight, doing more repetitions, resisting thicker bands (tubing), or by adding exercises to your routine.

How Do Muscles Get Stronger?

There are several theories regarding how muscles accomplish the cellular changes that lead to greater strength. The prevailing wisdom on this matter states that when the intensity is sufficient, strength training causes micro-tears in the muscle tissue (which may also account for soreness during early phases of strength training). After a standard strength-training workout, the micro-tears heal within 24 to 48 hours, and the muscle's performance capacity is then greater.

The 8–12 Double Variable Routine

The numbers 8 and 12 refer to repetitions, the term *double variable* refers to the two variables in your workout—the repetitions and the weight. Select a weight and see if you can perform eight repetitions (reps) with good form. If you do 8 repetitions properly, keep going. (If you cannot do 8 repetitions try a lighter weight.) If you can do more than 12 repetitions, stop after 12, take a rest of a minute or two, increase the weight slightly, and do another set. Continue in this manner until you find a weight you can lift at least 8 times, but not 13.

This weight will be your starting weight for the exercise you have been testing. After some period of time, you may find you are able to complete 12 repetitions with this weight. You may stay at that prescription (weight and reps) if you wish to maintain your strength. If you want to increase your strength you will increase the weight slightly. This additional weight may take your repetitions down—that's OK. You will gradually work your way back up to 12 repetitions.

This routine is a safe and effective way to begin a strength-training program. A basic routine will include squats, knee extension, knee flexion, heel raises, bent-arm row, seated row, military presses, bench presses, triceps extensions, curls, forearm curls, and abdominal work. After you are comfortable with this routine, you may want to try circuit training.

Circuit training involves a series of strength-training exercises of 12 to 15 repetitions, each using a moderate amount of weight. Circuit training can be performed most effectively on strength-training machines because you can preset the weight on the machine. If you have been training with the 8–12 Double Variable Routine, you already know your capabilities. In order to do the higher number of repetitions the likely adjustment you will have to make is lowering the weight on each machine by a plate or two. Once you begin the circuit you move quickly from one station to the next without stopping. The circuit should address at least eight major muscle groups. Ten stations is a typical circuit, but you can do as many as fifteen. To achieve exceptional muscular endurance go through your circuit once or twice more.

Thirty-second circuit training (30CT) is a variation in which you preset a moderate weight at each station and then do as many repetitions as you can in thirty seconds at each station; 30CT works well if you have a partner, a personal trainer, or a coach to time you at each station. It can also be used for a group of athletes whose strength levels are not too different. The stronger athletes will do more repetitions with the preset weight, but all participants start and finish at the same time.

• Frequency: Most of the research on strength training recommends 48 hours between workouts because it is important to let the muscles heal and recover. If you are going to add a full-body strength-training routine utilizing twelve major muscle groups to your weekly aerobic workouts, then you will be cross training for strength three times per week. With three such workouts per week you can expect to increase strength. There is evidence that strength can be maintained with two quality strength-training workouts per week.

If you are so fortunate as to have twenty to thirty minutes available each day, you could give yourself a program where you exercise your upper body and lower body on alternate days. For example, if your Monday, Wednesday, Friday aerobic exercise is powered by your legs, you would cross train for upper body strength on those days, and if you are after strength development in your legs (beyond what your aerobic workout is providing) you would do lower body strength training on Tuesdays, Thursdays, and Saturdays.

Again, rest is critical. Your muscles must recover from one workout before you work them hard again. If you begin a strength training workout and you can tell you "just don't have it," adjust your workout for that day and come back strong the next day.

• Duration: The duration of your strength-training workout depends on several factors:

- The time you spend warming up
- How many muscle groups you are going to train
- The number of repetitions you do per set
- The number of sets
- The amount of rest you take between sets
- Cooldown

With practice you will find you can complete a quality strength-training workout in about 25 minutes. Here is a sample breakdown for a time-efficient strength-training workout:

Joint readiness through stretching = 5 mins.

No. muscle groups = 10

No. repetitions per set = 8 at 6 seconds per rep =	48 sec.
(call it one minute per set)	
No. sets = 1 per muscle group = 10; 10 x 1 minute per set =	10 mins.
Rest between sets = 30 seconds x 9 =	4.5 mins.
Cooldown (stretching) =	5 mins.
Total workout time =	24.5 mins.

Most people training for strength use the same basic exercises. Both sides of the body should be developed equally and the opposing muscle or muscle group should be trained. For example, if you do knee extensions for your quadriceps, you must do knee flexion for your hamstrings (biceps femoris).

One exercise per muscle group will provide you with worthwhile results. Of course, if you are an advanced athlete in need of a very high level of strength you may need to do two, three, or four exercises per muscle group.

Your workout should be set up so that you use your largest muscles first and work your way down to the smaller muscles. Your largest muscles require the most energy and use the smaller muscles to assist during a given lift. If you have already exhausted the smaller muscles, you will find it difficult to handle enough weight to exercise the larger muscle groups properly.

A typical sequence applying the concept of moving from large to small muscle groups is:

1. Hips and lower back
2. Lower body: quadriceps, hamstrings, calves
3. Torso: back, shoulders, chest
4. Arms: triceps, biceps, forearms
5. Abdominals

For functional fitness and recreational sports performance the 8–12 Double Variable Routine described earlier is excellent and time-efficient. However, if you wish to concentrate specifically on gaining greater strength, experts suggest you test yourself for your one-repetition maximum (as explained on page 81) at each strength-training exercise and do the following:

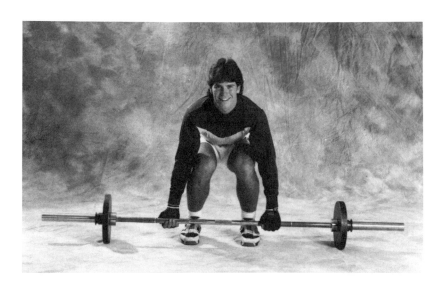

The Dead Lift Starting Position

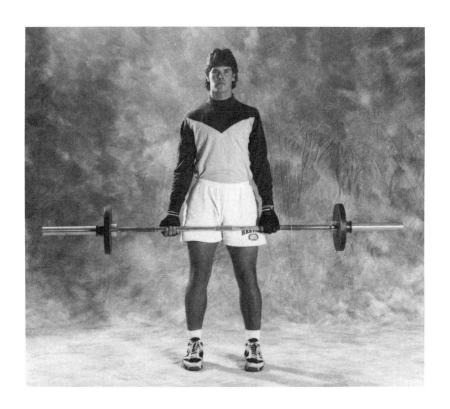

The Dead Lift Finish Position

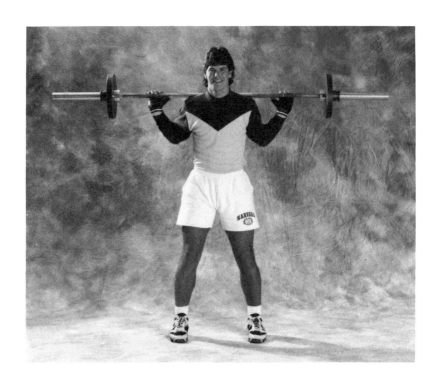

The Squat Starting Position

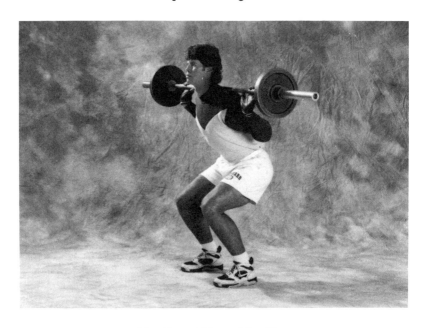

The Squat Flexed Position

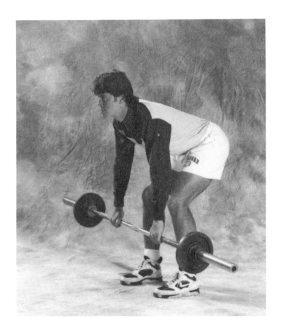

Bent Over Row Start Position

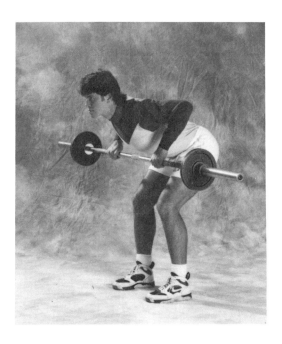

Bent Over Row Finish Position

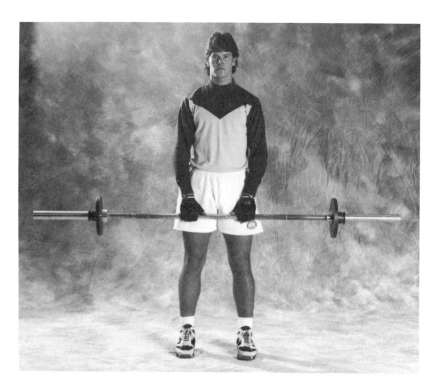

Upright Row Start Position

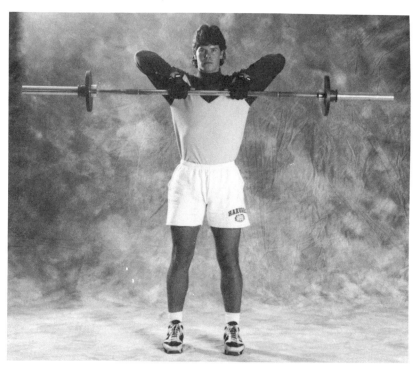

Upright Row Finish Position

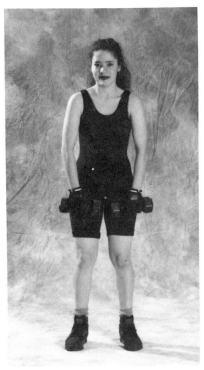 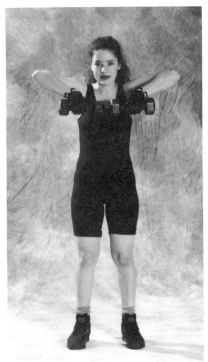

Upright Rowing performed with dumbbells.   Finish Position
Starting Position

Cross Training for Strength

- - - - - - - - - - - - - - -

Weight   = 85% of 1 rep max
No. repetitions = 1 to 5
No. sets   = 4 to 8

If you want to concentrate on muscular endurance, this workout should be effective: **Cross Training for Muscular Endurance**

Weight   = 50% of 1 rep max
No. repetitions = 20 to 50
No. sets   = 2 to 4

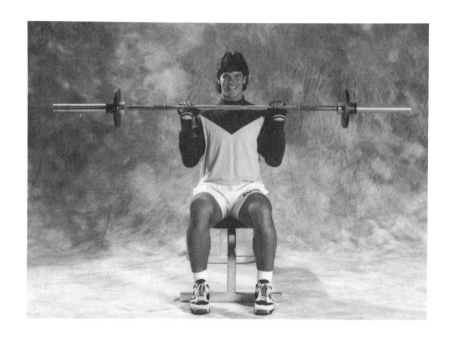

Military Press Starting Position

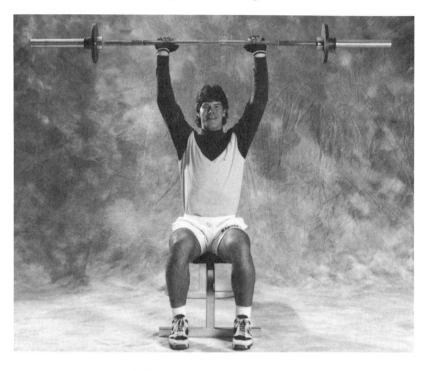

Military Press Finish Position

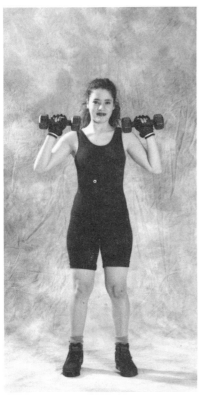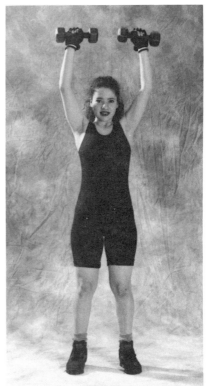

Military Press performed with dumbbells.
5A = Starting Position
5B = Finish Position

Whether you set up your strength-training workout to work toward functional fitness, absolute strength, or exceptional muscular endurance, remember that you should increase only one variable at a time. Usually you would first increase repetitions, then sets, and then the number of exercises.

Two of the most popular weight-training machine systems are variable resistance and isokinetic. With variable resistance equipment the weight in the stack you are lifting remains constant, but the leverage change in the machine makes the resistance greater at some joint angles. The purpose of variable resistance equipment is to keep the muscles fully loaded throughout the full range of motion.

True isokinetic equipment limits the speed at which the

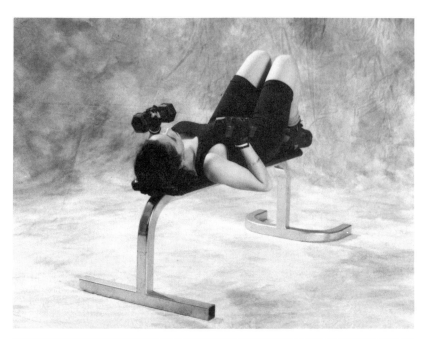

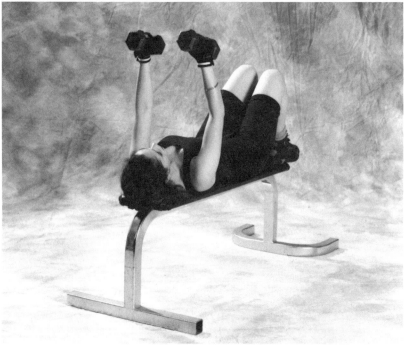

The Bench Press performed with dumbbells.
Starting Position
Finish Position

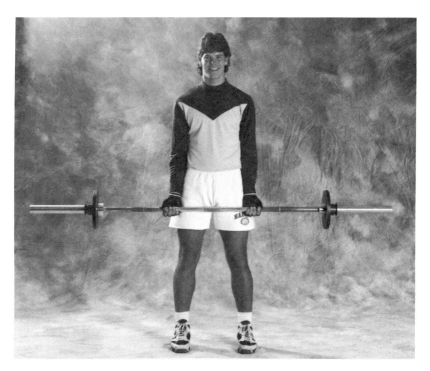

Biceps Curl Starting Position

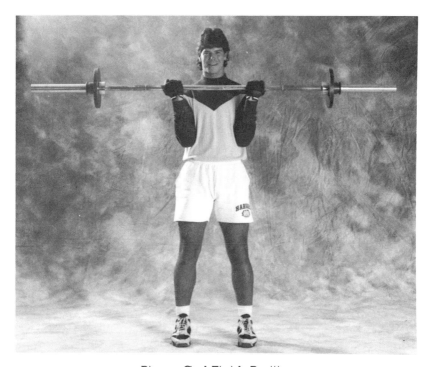

Biceps Curl Finish Position

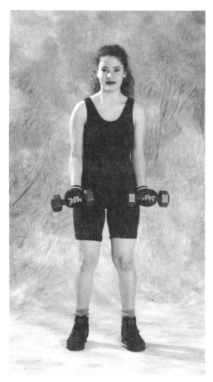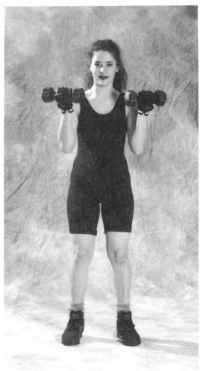

The Biceps Curl performed with dumbbells.   Finish Position
Starting Position

exercise machine will move. This is a safety feature because it allows a muscle to contract at its maximum force
from full extension to full contraction without accelerating.
Isokinetic equipment is often used during rehabilitation
programs for injured muscles.

Weak Stomach and a Bad Back?
Train Your Abdominal Muscles

Abdominal exercises give you a terrific return on a
benefits-per-minute basis. As mentioned earlier, maintaining good abdominal strength is one of the best ways to
prevent lower back pain. Weak abdominals (and inflex-
ible hamstrings) allow the pelvis to tilt forward, causing
lordosis, or curvature in the lower back. This places in-

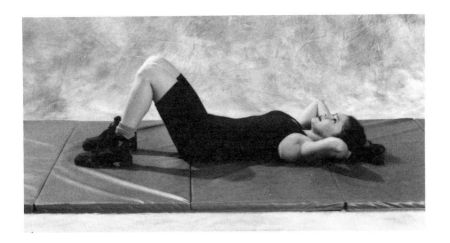

Abdominal Curl Starting Position

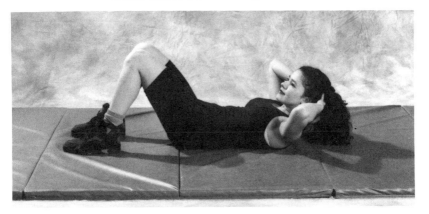

Abdominal Curl Flexed Position

creased pressure on the vertebral column and the other postural muscles, causing the muscles to fatigue and eventually leading to a problem known as "lower-back pain syndrome." Lower back pain is the number one symptomatic complaint expressed to physicians by patients 25 to 60 years old. (Chapter 6 includes a test you can do at home to assess your hamstring flexibility.)

If you can, it's good to begin your "Strong Stomach—Healthy Back" workout with five minutes of light aerobic exercise as described in Chapter 3, followed by the stretches below. (If you want to do this workout at home but do not have aerobic exercise equipment just begin with the stretches and go slowly. The stretches are described in Chapter 4.)

- Upper back
- Lateral trunk
- Lower back
- Lower back, gluteus maximus, hips
- Lower back and hamstrings
- Hamstrings

There are four muscle groups in the abdominal area: rectus abdominus, internal oblique, external oblique, and the transversalis. The exercises described here engage each of these muscle groups. You may begin by doing two or three repetitions of each exercise. Rest as needed between exercises. As you find your abdominal strength increasing you can work your way up to five or ten repetitions per exercise.

Toning Muscles With Straps, Bands, or Tubing

Straps, bands, or tubing are being used successfully by exercisers to develop and maintain muscle tone. These devices can provide a legitimate muscle toning workout by providing resistance against a given muscle group. Their popularity is increasing rapidly with personal trainers and their clients because they cost less than a set of free weights and take up much less space. These devices are terrific for anyone who is traveling. If you have a business trip or a vacation coming up, just pack one of these lightweight devices and you can continue your muscle toning exercise wherever you are.

Lifeline is one such system that uses tubing and is highly recommended by New York City personal trainers (Lifeline, 1421 S. Park Street, Madison, WI 53715; 1-800-553-6633). Dynabands is another version being used as an alternative to traditional strength training (order through Fitness Wholesale, 3064 W. Edgerton, Silver Lake, Ohio 44224).

Abdominal Workout

Try to follow the instructions and mimic the sketches to the best of your ability because form is important. Doing the abdominal exercises properly will give you the maximum return for your effort. Each exercise should be performed in a slow and controlled manner.

Your abdominal muscles will respond well to working in different positions and to multiple repetitions. There are many abdominal exercise combinations which will provide improved muscle tone and help reduce the risk of lower back problems. The exercises explained on the following pages are presented in order of difficulty, more or less. Here is a sample workout which progresses on a weekly basis.

Week One: Do any five exercises three times each (5 x 3 = 15). Add one exercise per week until you are doing all ten (10 x 3 = 30). Then, over a period of time, add one repetition per exercise until you can do ten repetitions of each exercise (10 x 10 = 100).

Side Bend

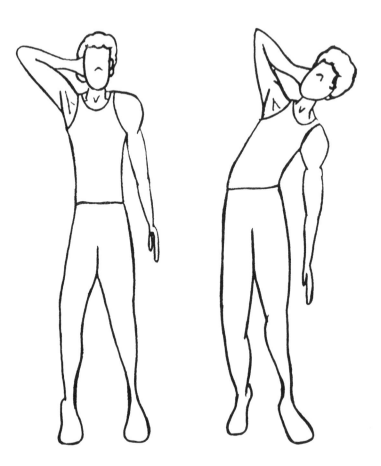

Stand with feet shoulder width apart. Place one hand on the side of your head and slowly lower the opposite arm towards the ground. After completing desired repetitions, switch hand positions and work opposite side. Holding a weight of two to ten pounds (or more if you are able) in the down hand will increase the effectiveness of this exercise.

Double-Knee Twist

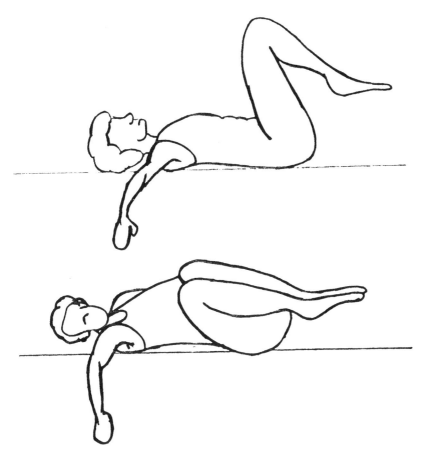

Lie on your back with arms extended away from your body and knees flexed up over your chest. Slowly lower both legs to one side such that they are within two to three inches of the floor. Bring both legs back to starting position, then repeat movement to other side.

Curl

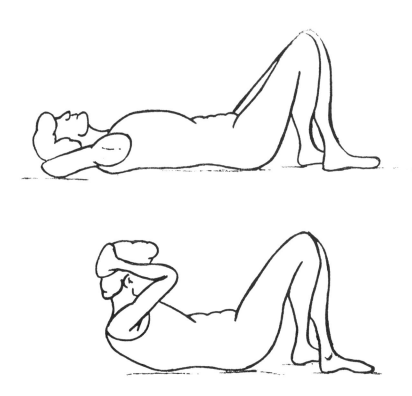

Lie on your back, knees bent, feet flat, hands clasped gently behind head. Slowly curl up bringing your head and shoulder blades off the floor. Lower your body slowly back to starting position.

Hip Flexion

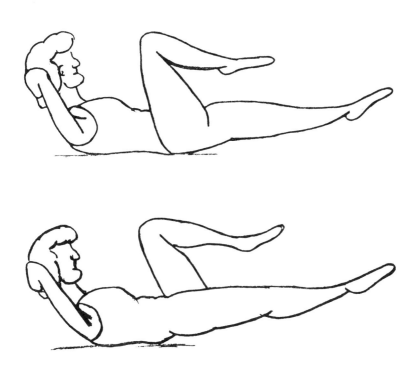

Slowly curl your head and shoulders off floor while bringing one flexed knee towards your head. Lower your upper body and leg back to starting position. Repeat using opposite leg in same manner.

Partial Curl

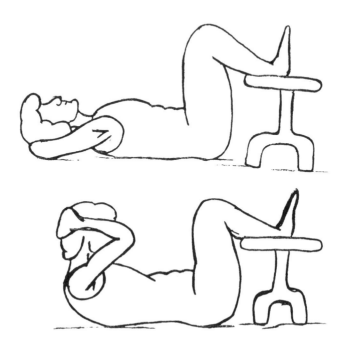

Lie on a carpet or mat, rest calves over a bench or chair with hands clasped gently behind your head. Slowly curl body so that elbows move towards knees. Return to starting position and repeat.

Lying Curl

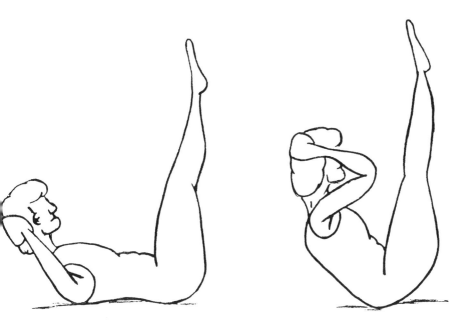

Lie on back, hands clasped gently behind head, legs together pointing up. Lift head and shoulders three to four inches off the floor. Then curl up bringing elbows and head towards knees. Return to starting position and repeat.

Bent-Knee Sit-Up

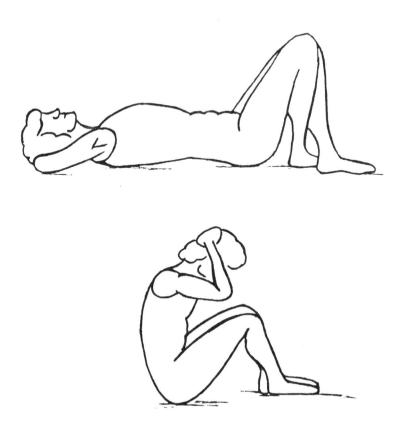

Lie on your back with knees bent and clasp hands gently behind head. Slowly curl up until elbows are close to or touching knees. Do not pull on your head. Slowly return to starting position and repeat.

Double Curl

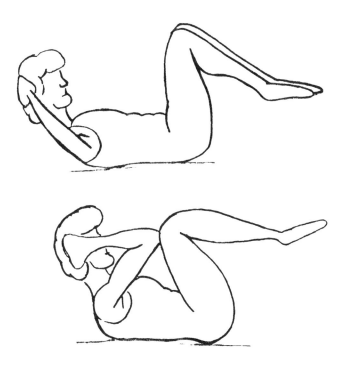

Lie on your back with your shoulder blades just off the floor. Lift your legs and bend your knees at a 90 degree angle. Curl your upper and lower body at the same time until your knees touch your elbows. Slowly return to starting position and repeat.

Bicycle Curl

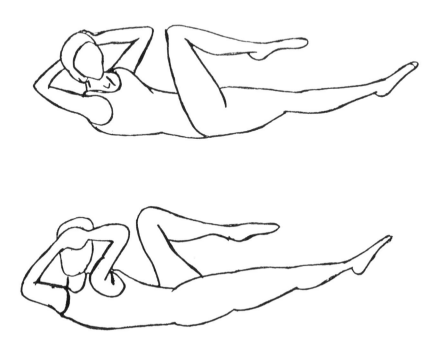

Lie on your back with hands clasped gently behind your head. Pull your head and shoulders gently off the floor. From this starting position twist your torso and bring one knee up so that the opposite knee and elbow will touch. Slowly lower your upper body and leg to starting position and repeat with other elbow and knee.

Pop-Ups

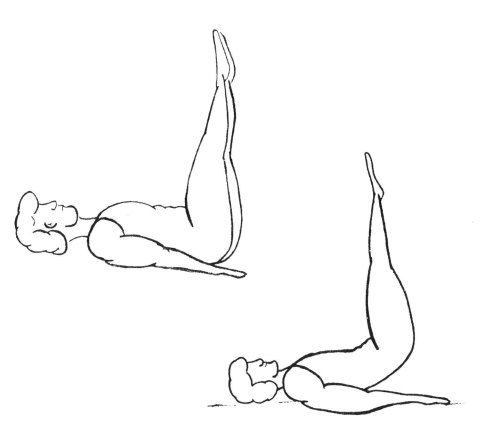

Lie on your back with hands alongside hips and legs pointed straight up, knees just slightly flexed. Lift hips up off ground three to four inches. Slowly lower hips to start position. Repeat.

Manual Resistance Training

The resistance in manual training is provided by a training partner. Your partner will need to be familiar with the techniques involved in this method of toning muscles and should not be drastically different from you in strength. Manual resistance training has been used by U.S. armed forces stationed overseas (far from any exercise equipment). It can be effective because your muscles respond equally well to an overload whether the resistance is provided by dumbbells, barbells, weight stacks, tubing, or your partner's resistance.

For example, to work your shoulder muscles with manual resistance you would sit down on the floor with your palms just outside your shoulders facing up. Your partner would stand behind you and place his hands on top of yours. On your signal you will begin pressing up while your partner presses down. Gradually your partner allows you to extend your arms above your head (just as you would for the military press). Dan Riley's book *Maximum Muscular Fitness* (West Point, NY: Leisure Press, 1982) clearly explains thirty-one manual resistance exercises.

The Gravitron

The Gravitron is a machine that allows you to do several different exercises which develop upper body strength in just a few minutes. You step on to a platform and input your body weight on a computer console. Then you program the Gravitron so that you will work (lift) against a percentage of your body weight. For example, if you weigh 130 pounds and you can normally do only one pull-up, you can program the Gravitron for a 50% body weight workout. The hydraulic unit under the platform will provide 65 pounds of force upwards and suddenly you are doing pull-ups with half your body weight! Lifting 65 pounds, you find you can do ten pull-ups—a much better workout for you. Then you go on to do wide-grip pull-ups to work your lattisimus dorsi muscles, and then a set of dips for

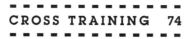

your triceps and deltoids, and in three minutes you have accomplished a terrific upper-body strength training work-out.

Fitness centers and health clubs are adding gravitrons to their strength training circuits all across the United States.

6

Assessing Your Physical Fitness Needs

I n their book *Concepts of Physical Fitness* (William C. Brown Publishers, 1991) Corbin and Lindsay describe physical fitness as "the entire human organism's ability to function efficiently and effectively. Physical fitness is associated with a person's ability to work effectively, to enjoy leisure time, to be healthy, to resist disease, and to meet emergency situations. Though the development of physical fitness is the result of many things, optimal physical fitness is not possible without regular exercise."

Cross training develops optimal physical fitness, but it is important to know what your current level of physical fitness is before you alter or expand your exercise routine. Before evaluating your physical fitness, let your doctor know what you are planning. Medical screening may be advisable depending on your current health and family history.

Save your test results on a copy of the Physical Fitness Assessment form provided at the end of this chapter so you will be able to see your progress after cross training.

The Step Test

1. Prior to taking the Step Test, stretch your hamstrings and quadriceps gently (see chapter 4). Then sit quietly for a few minutes to be sure your heart is at its resting rate.
2. Step up and down on a twelve-inch bench for three minutes at a rate of twenty-four steps per minute. One step consists of four beats, that is, "up with the left foot, up with the right foot, down with the left foot, down with the right foot."
3. Immediately after the exercise, sit down on the bench and relax. Don't talk.
4. Locate your pulse.
5. Five seconds after the exercise ends, begin counting your pulse. Count your pulse for sixty seconds.
6. Your score is your sixty-second pulse count (heart rate). Locate your score and your rating on the table below.
7. Cool down and repeat the hamstring and quadriceps stretches.

Step Test Rating Scale

Classification	Sixty-Second Heart Rate
High Performance Zone	84 or less
Good Fitness Zone	85–95
Marginal (or Fair) Zone	96–119
Low (or Poor) Zone	120 and above

The 12-Minute Run

1. Locate an area where a specific distance is already marked, such as a school track. Or measure a

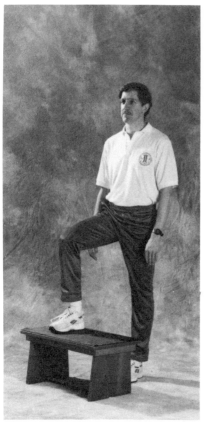
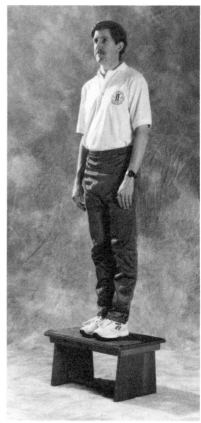
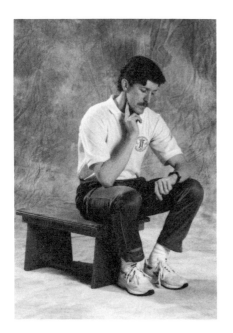

Upon completion of the
Three-Minute Step Test you sit
down and count your pulse
for one minute.

specific distance using a bicycle or automobile odometer.
2. Use a stopwatch or wristwatch to time a 12-minute period.
3. For best results, warm up prior to the test, then run at a steady pace for the entire 12 minutes (cool down by walking slowly after you have completed the test).
4. Determine the distance you can run in 12 minutes in fractions of a mile.
5. Locate your score and rating, according to your age, on the table below.

12-Minute Run Test (Scores in Miles)

Men			
Classification (age) 17–26	27–39	40–49	50+
High Performance 1.80+	1.60+	1.50+	1.40+
Good Fitness Zone 1.55–1.79	1.45–1.59	1.40–1.49	1.25–1.39
Marginal Zone 1.35–1.54	1.30–1.44	1.25–1.39	1.10–1.24
Low (Poor) Zone Less than 1.35	Less than 1.30	Less than 1.25	Less than 1.10

Women			
Classification (age) 17–26	27–39	40–49	50+
High Performance 1.45+	1.35+	1.25+	1.15+
Good Fitness 1.25–1.44	1.20–1.34	1.15–1.24	1.05–1.14
Marginal Zone 1.15–1.24	1.05–1.19	1.00–1.14	0.95–1.04
Low (Poor) Zone Less than 1.15	Less than 1.05	Less than 1.00	Less than .95

Flexibility Testing

Flexibility is specific to the joint and attached muscles being tested. With lower back pain accounting for more missed work days in the United States than any ailment except respiratory illness, it's important to know if you need to be stretching your hamstrings and lower back more regularly. The following test evaluates the flexibility of these two muscle groups.

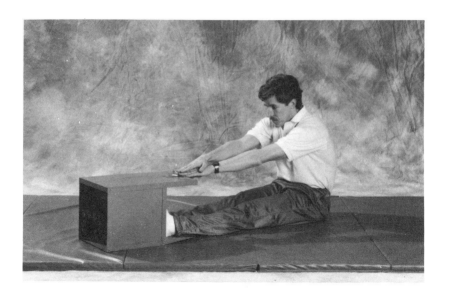

To assess your hamstring and lower back flexibility do this simple Sit & Reach Flexibility Test which can be conducted with a yardstick and a box.

Sit and Reach Test

Sit with your legs extended directly in front of you and with the backs of your knees pressed against the floor. Your stocking feet (no sneakers) should be placed up against a box to which a yardstick has been attached. The yardstick should be on top of the box with the lower measurement close to you, and the six-inch mark placed at the point where your foot contacts the box. Place your hands one on top of the other and, keeping your hands together, slowly reach forward as far as possible, *without* bending your knees. Note the distance you reached on the yardstick.

Find your score on the scale below to determine your flexibility rating.

Flexibility Rating Scale (In Inches)

	Men	Women
High Performance	14+	15+
Good Fitness	10–13.9	10–14.9
Marginal Zone	6–9.9	6–9
Low (Poor) Zone	Less than 6	Less than 6

Shoulder Flexibility Test

1. Raise your right arm, bend your elbow, and reach down across your back as far as possible.
2. At the same time, extend your left arm down and behind your back, bend your elbow up across your back, and try to stretch your hands until they meet or overlap.
3. Measure the distance to the nearest half-inch. If your fingers overlap, you are scoring in positive figures; if they just touch, you are scoring at zero; if they fail to meet, you are scoring in negative figures.

Bench Press Test

As for flexibility, strength is also specific to the muscle group being tested. The correlation between strength for a major muscle group and the other major muscle groups has been estimated at 80%. The Bench Press Test utilizes the pectoral and triceps muscles to evaluate upper body strength. The rating charts on pages 82 and 83 are based on the universal dynamic variable resistance bench press resistance machine.

1. Men should set the pin to their approximate bodyweight. Women should set the pin at the first plate.
2. For each lift, be sure to exhale as you press up.
3. After each successful lift move the pin so the next lift will be with more weight. Your goal is to find your maximum lift capability within five or six lifts.

Absolute Strength
1 Repetition Maximum Bench Press

- -

$$\text{Bench Press Weight Ratio} = \frac{\text{Weight Pushed in Lbs.}}{\text{Body Weight in Lbs.}}$$

MALE

AGE

%	<20	20–29	30–39	40–49	50–59	60+	
99	>1.76	>1.63	>1.35	>1.20	>1.05	>.94	S
95	1.76	1.63	1.35	1.20	1.05	.94	
90	1.46	1.48	1.24	1.10	.97	.89	
85	1.38	1.37	1.17	1.04	.93	.84	E
80	1.34	1.32	1.12	1.00	.90	.82	
75	1.29	1.26	1.08	.96	.87	.79	
70	1.24	1.22	1.04	.93	.84	.77	G
65	1.23	1.18	1.01	.90	.81	.74	
60	1.19	1.14	.98	.88	.79	.72	
55	1.16	1.10	.96	.86	.77	.70	
50	1.13	1.06	.93	.84	.75	.68	F
45	1.10	1.03	.90	.82	.73	.67	
40	1.06	.99	.88	.80	.71	.65	
35	1.01	.96	.86	.78	.70	.65	
30	.96	.93	.83	.76	.68	.63	P
25	.93	.90	.81	.74	.66	.60	
20	.89	.88	.78	.72	.63	.57	
15	.86	.84	.75	.69	.60	.56	
10	.81	.80	.71	.650	.57	.53	VP
5	.76	.72	.65	.590	.53	.49	
1	<.76	<.72	<.65	<.590	<.53	<.49	

S = superior   E = excellent   G = good   F = fair   P = poor   VP = very poor

Absolute Strength
1 Repetition Maximum Bench Press

- -

$$\text{Bench Press Weight Ratio} = \frac{\text{Weight Pushed in Lbs.}}{\text{Body Weight in Lbs.}}$$

Female

Age

%	>20	20–29	30–39	40–49	50–59	60+	
99	>.88	>1.01	>.82	>.77	>.68	>.72	S
95	.88	1.01	.82	.77	.68	.72	
90	.83	.90	.76	.71	.61	.64	
85	.81	.83	.72	.66	.57	.59	E
80	.77	.80	.70	.62	.55	.54	
75	.76	.77	.65	.60	.53	.53	
70	.64	.74	.63	.57	.52	.51	G
65	.70	.72	.62	.55	.50	.48	
60	.65	.70	.60	.54	.48	.46	
55	.64	.68	.58	.53	.47	.46	
50	.63	.65	.57	.52	.46	.45	F
45	.60	.63	.55	.51	.45	.44	
40	.57	.59	.53	.50	.44	.43	
35	.56	.58	.52	.48	.43	.41	
30	.56	.56	.51	.47	.42	.40	P
25	.55	.53	.49	.45	.41	.39	
20	.53	.51	.47	.43	.39	.39	
15	.52	.50	.45	.42	.38	.36	
10	.50	.480	.42	.38	.37	.33	VP
5	.41	.436	.39	.35	.305	.26	
1	<.41	<.436	<.39	<.35	<.305	<.26	

S = superior   E = excellent   G = good   F = fair   P = poor   VP = very poor

(Bench Press tables reprinted by permission. The Cooper Institute for Aerobics Research, Dallas, Texas.)

Physical Fitness Assessment

Date: _____   Retest date: _____

Aerobic Capacity

Classification

Step Test Recovery Heart Rate = _____   _____

12:00 run time = _____   _____

Flexibility

Sit & Reach score = _____   _____

Shoulder flexibility test

    fingers: overlap _____ (good)

        touch _____ (acceptable)

        don't touch _____ (need to improve)

Strength

Maximum lift = _____ lbs.

Bench Press Ratio (max. lift/body weight) = _____   _____

Physical fitness goals: _____

_____

Cross training options: _____

_____

7

Selecting
Your Cross-Training
Activity

The three foremost questions to consider as you begin thinking about selecting your cross-training activity are:

1. Which benefits of cross training are you looking for?
2. Of your options, which will best provide the benefits you seek?
3. Which of your cross-training options are practical?

As you go through this chapter, try to keep an open mind. When you have finished reading it you will have a good sense of the factors involved in selecting a cross-training activity. By thinking about these factors you will be able to make your selection with confidence that it will work for you.

Cross Training During Injury Rehabilitation

If you are cross training during injury rehabilitation then you are going to select an activity that allows the injured area to heal. If you are cross training to *prevent* overuse injuries, you will be wise to select an activity that does not involve the muscle groups of your primary activity or else uses those muscle groups in a much different range of motion. For example, squash is not the best cross-training alternative for the lifelong tennis player with elbow pain. But this tennis player might do well to look at running (and sprint workouts), step machines, or aerobic dance classes because these cross-training activities offer a way to maintain conditioning while the injured elbow heals.

Cross Training to Develop Overall Physical Fitness

If you want to cross train because you would like to develop overall physical fitness, you can work with your physical fitness assessment results from chapter 6. Let's assume your areas for improvement are upper and lower body flexibility and upper body strength. Swimming would be one of the best cross training options since it provides upper body flexibility and upper body muscular development (see page 178). Or you might want to add a flexibility routine and strength-training routine to your workout. If you have the time and appropriate access you could add an activity such as cross-country skiing. With a cross-country ski machine you can work on your physical fitness needs year-round.

Cross Training for Variety

If you are cross training for variety you are in a great situation. Ask yourself, What would I like to do? What looks like fun? Is there an activity or sport I have been thinking about trying?

Now's the time to do it.

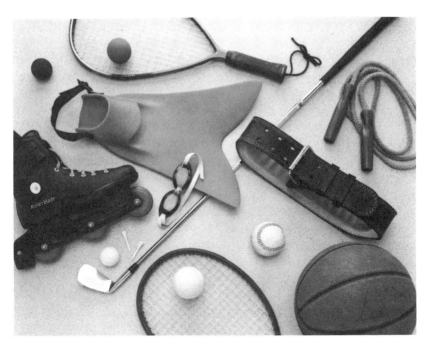

Variety is one of the great benefits of cross training.

Cross Training for the Challenge

How about cross training for the challenge and sense of accomplishment? Select an activity that appeals to you. Maybe it's in-line skating—rent a pair of skates and check it out. Or dancing, you never learned the polka, so sign up for a few lessons with your partner and soon you will dance across the floor without even thinking about the calories you are burning.

Cross Training to Make New Friends

To make new friends, select a cross-training activity done in a group setting, such as aerobic indoor exercise in a fitness center or a health club. Or select an activity conducted in a class with ongoing lessons. Chapter 11 subsections, "Never Let Them See You Sweat" and "Dance To Your Heart's Content" both discuss activities offered with lessons.

Cross Training to Strengthen a Relationship

To strengthen a relationship through cross training, the two people must be willing to sit down and come to an agreement on an activity they would like to do together. This process could begin by each person making a list of ten activities they are ready to try. They would then compare the two lists and see if any activity is on both lists. If so, the couple is on their way to strengthening their relationship through cross training. Next, together they should review the how, where, and when of the new activity. If they pick paddleball, for example, they would have to answer several questions. Where are the courts and when are they available? Are there fees involved? Are there children to be cared for while they play? What's the best time of day to play?

If you value the relationship, be willing to think through these questions so that you and your partner can have some fun and be physically fit together. You will find your planning to be well worth the effort in the long run.

Cross Training in New Locations

Are you willing to expand your exercise horizons? If so you may find that you can do some great workouts in a new environment. How about planning a vacation around an activity like hiking? (see chapter 11.)

Cross Training to Open
New Time-of-Day Workout Options

Have you thought about how much time you have available for cross training? Not as much as you would like, you say—but wait a minute. Take a look at these time-management cross-training workout ideas and perhaps you will find one or two that will work for you.

Destination Workouts

Can you use either your primary form of exercise or your cross-training activity to get you to your destination? In other words, can you walk, jog, run, cycle, skate, ski, or hike to your destination? Let's assume you are ready to explore riding a bike to work and home a few times a week. You still need to check into a few things. What route will you take as you ride to work? How long will it take? (In some urban areas cycling is faster than mass transit.) Where will you put your bike at work? If you ride long enough to break a sweat, can you find a place to get washed up and change into your work clothes? After you have the answers to these questions, you are ready to add destination workouts to your cross-training program.

Morning Madness

Some would say it is mad to suggest exercise in the morning, but it can be done. If your cross-training need is balanced physical fitness, you may be able to accomplish that goal by doing simple calisthenics for fifteen minutes three times per week. Or, if you need to improve your flexibility, use the fifteen minutes just to stretch. All you have to do is set the alarm clock 20 minutes earlier, do your exercises consistently, and you will be cross training successfully.

Lunchtime Latitude

What kind of latitude do you have at lunchtime? Are you at work or at home for lunch? Are there any exercise facilities or locker room facilities near you? If you answer yes to the last question, perhaps you should reexamine your lunch hour with an eye for adding a cross-training workout. If you think you will need an hour and 15 minutes altogether, maybe the boss is open to flex-time. You could either start 15 minutes earlier each day you work out, or stay 15 minutes later. Or, could you take two 45 minute lunches and two 75 minute (workout) lunches each week? Try to come up with a plan that will allow you to add your cross-training workouts to the middle of your day.

Negotiating Weekends

If you are in a serious relationship, or married and there are children, too, you may have to negotiate for cross-training time on the weekends. These negotiations may take many forms, but there is one premise you might put up front: Exercising and cross training are good for your physical and mental well-being; therefore, your partner should support your efforts to work out. Your partner's reward comes from seeing you healthier, more fit, and happier. Perhaps your partner will go and do a workout when you are done with yours.

You will both, of course, then show your appreciation for getting to cross train on the weekends by doing your fair share of the errands, chores, etc.

Family Fitness

If your weekends are your own, you should be able to find time to cross train sometime between Friday night and Monday morning, or if you work weekends, on your days off. You can guide the family toward training and fitness by scheduling special events around some type of activity.

Many health clubs have exercise classes for adults and children going on at the same time. Or, if the kids are too young, there may be a child care area for junior while you cross train nearby.

How about skating together? Or going out for a family bike ride? Or a day trip climbing hills? Children as young as six can cross-country ski on a beginner's trail. Maybe a simple family walk in a park would be a good start.

A Night Out with the Boys (or Girls)

What do you do on a typical night out with your best buddies? Watch a ball game? Play cards, have dessert, or just chat? Whatever it may be, how about considering the idea of a social outing organized around some type of exercise? At the next get-together bring it up for discussion. If you can get a consensus on *what* to do, then you can move right to logistics. If there are too many different preferences, try taking turns—one week one sport, the next week try someone else's preference.

What's Best for You?

Other factors involved in evaluating which cross training activity is best for you are personality, body type, and athletic requirements.

Personality

It is important that your personality fit your activity. For example, when President Gerald Lynch arrives at John Jay College each day he knows he will have a constant stream of meetings, appointments, and special events. He discovered years ago that his best primary activity was running to work through Central Park because he needs that thirty minutes in the morning for himself. When he has time, he cross trains by riding a stationary bike (he reads his mail at the same time) and he does strength training.

If you are alone during most of your workday but are gregarious by nature, you might enjoy a cross-training option such as a step aerobics class, which will let you socialize with other exercises.

How do you feel about competition? NBA star and avid golfer Michael Jordan is a good example of a cross-training athlete who loves to compete at every opportunity. If you like to compete from within the framework of a team, there are plenty of options. If you would rather rely on your own ability, you will want to choose sports that offers one-on-one confrontations.

Body Type

The world of exercise welcomes all body types and there are cross-training activities for everyone. The significance of body type lies mostly in the areas of injury potential and probability of success in certain sports. If perchance you are carrying a few extra pounds you may find non-weight-bearing cross-training activities easier on your joints. Consider the options of swimming, cycling, indoor rowing machines, or low-impact aerobic dance classes (no jumping; you keep one foot on the floor at all times.)

Generalizations can always be made about the body type needed for success in a particular sport, but exceptions can be found. Most of the best basketball players are usually fairly tall, but look at NBA players Tyrone Bogues (5′ 3″), Spud Webb (5′ 7″), and Michael Adams (5′ 10″). The best gymnasts tend to be compact and of average or below average height, but Tim Daggett (over 6′) had a terrific collegiate gymnastic career and competed for the United States as an Olympic gymnast.

Cross training will let you change certain aspects of your body so that you can become more successful in your sport. Can cross training affect a basketball player's or a gymnast's height? Afraid not. But you can reduce your percent age of body fat through aerobic cross training, and in many sports your performance is enhanced by being lean. If you are doing a sport like martial arts, which requires muscular endurance, strength training will help you.

Athletic Requirements

Just about anyone can cross train with any activity or sport. Women are taking boxing classes these days because they like the conditioning and the ability to defend themselves. Men of all sizes are found in aerobic dance classes because they like the challenge of learning the steps and the excellent workout they get. If you are very competitive be aware that certain sports have specific physical requirements for superior physical performance. You can get a fine workout from cross training with a racquet sport like squash, but if your hand-eye coordination is only fair, be advised you may be on the short end of a lot of matches for a while. The solution is to find opponents of approximately equal ability so you will be able to enjoy a competitive and fair match.

What's Practical?: Cost and Convenience

Spending money so that you and your family can cross train is the best investment you will ever make. You will be healthier, more fit, and happier. Whatever you can afford, consider the cost an investment in your well-being.

The more convenient your cross-training options are, the better your chances of staying with them over a period of time. Consider purchasing home exercise equipment so that you will be able to exercise more easily and gain cross-training benefits at the same time. Aerobic cross-training options include indoor cross-country ski machines, rowing machines, step machines, treadmills, stationary bikes, slide boards, and jump ropes. Strength training can be done at home with a barbell/dumbbell set, with calisthenics, through bands, or by manual resistance exercises.

Chapters 8 and 9 address the reader who has selected a favorite sport and is familiar with its basics. You will learn how to gain the benefits of cross training for your sport, not how to play the game or how to be a runner.

If you select classic cross training, you will find that chapter 10 on the triathlon tells you all you need to know about training for each of the three components.

If you need cross-training ideas, twenty choices that can be enjoyed without competition are analyzed and introduced in chapter 11, "Cross Training with Activities." Referring to the Physical Fitness Benefits chart for any given activity will tell you whether that activity complements your primary form of exercise.

8

Cross Training
for Sport

For improved athletic performance in any of the fourteen competitive sports discussed in this chapter it's important to remember that you cross train as a supplement to sport-specific training.

Specificity of training, as discussed in chapter 3, is a principle of exercise that applies to success in sports. Adaptions in your metabolic, physiologic, and neuromuscular systems are directly dependent on the type of training you do. Therefore, to improve performance in any activity involving movement, you must perform the specific movement involved repeatedly. The more complicated the pattern of movement, the more critical it is that it be repeated precisely. The world of sports has a word for this concept: *practice*. You practice until you get it right, because repetition is a key to learning movement skills.

World-famous basketball player Earvin "Magic"

Johnson applied the principles of specificity of training to his extremely successful cross-training program with enormous results.

In the spring of 1991, just after Magic was diagnosed as having the AIDS virus, he announced that it would not be wise for him to attempt to play the entire grueling 82-game season of the National Basketball Association. The frequency of the games and the travel demands would lead to a cumulative fatigue that might be detrimental to his health. At the same time Magic's medical advisers told him that he could play safely in an exhibition game if he properly prepared his body through physical conditioning and rested well between training sessions. Knowing this, but unable to practice with his Los Angeles Laker teammates, Magic's solution was to design a cross-training program that would allow him to be ready to play in the 1992 NBA All-Star game.

Magic's program called for running, jumping, and weight lifting to prepare his body for the cardiovascular and muscular demands of an NBA game. Even though there are no weights to lift during a basketball game, the pushing and shoving of the inside game of the NBA involve gross motor movements with large muscle groups. For instance, the bench press exercise is useful to a professional basketball player because it develops the pectoral (chest) muscles needed to fight through a Charles Oakley pick.

Magic also trained by working on the *skills* specific to his sport. During this skill training Magic did ball-handling drills to keep his dribbling ability sharp and shooting drills to keep his shooting eye on target—to have "the touch," as basketball players say. Then he played half-court games so he could apply his conditioning and skills to game situations.

If Magic had done the running, jumping, and weight lifting without practicing his skills he would have lost the ball when he tried to dribble. If he had practiced shooting but did not do his running, within a matter of minutes he would have been unable to keep up with the pace of play at the NBA level. In fact, Magic did get slightly winded during the first quarter of the 1992 NBA All-Star game and he took a short rest. But he soon returned to the action at full speed, putting on a brilliant display of shooting and passing that culminated in his selection as the game's Most Valuable Player.

You can learn from Magic's cross-training success as you strive to improve your performance in your favorite sport. Analyze your sport by breaking it down into its components, and then review your training program. Are you addressing each component or have you been ignoring some aspect of your sport? When tennis star Chris Evert-Lloyd realized she was tiring too quickly and losing points because she couldn't get to the ball, it caused her to upgrade her cardiovascular training and helped her succeed against other highly fit opponents.

If your sport is baseball or softball, what happens when you hit the ball on the ground to the left side of the infield? Are you an automatic out because you are slow running to first base? What about working on getting a quick jump out of the batter's box and cross training with sprints of 90 feet?

Fourteen sports are discussed in this chapter. If your sport is here you will see what fitness benefits it provides. Combine this information with your own analysis of your sport's components, incorporate the principles of exercise, and you will be able to develop an appropriate cross-training program that will help you improve.

If your favorite sport is not included you can still cross train. Read through a section that discusses another sport with which you are familiar and you will learn the cross-training concepts. Then apply the concepts to your sport and begin working toward balanced physical fitness and better performance.

Cross Training for Sport
to Achieve Physical Fitness Balance

What if you are satisfied with your performance in competitive situations? What if you do not wish to put in hours of practice drills to fine-tune your skills yet feel your sport is lacking when it comes to providing complete physical

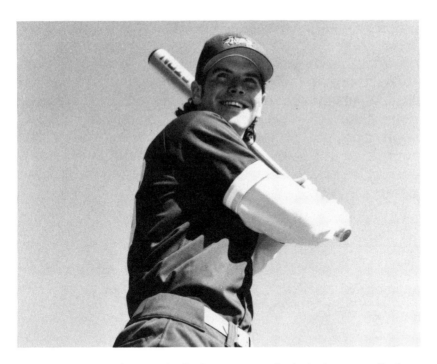

The most successful baseball players cross train to improve their strength, speed and quickness.

fitness? Look closely at the Physical Fitness Benefits chart for your sport to learn exactly which aspects of fitness you are missing. Then select an appropriate cross-training activity that will round out your physical fitness profile.

Cross Training for Baseball

In 1839 Abner Doubleday laid out the dimensions of the first baseball field in Cooperstown, New York. But it is Alexander Cartwright who is credited with the set of rules (for his Knickerbocker Base Ball Club) that changed what had been a child's pastime into a robust adult game. Although Cartwright's rules were adopted in 1845, it was ten years before baseball gained momentum. By the end of the 1850s hundreds of teams were taking the field in various cities. The first completely professional team was the Cincinnati Red Stockings, and the highest-paid player earned $1,400 for a forty-game season, or $35 per game. Today there are many major league baseball players with contracts paying over one million dollars per season. Nevertheless, "America's Game," as baseball is known, is still played for the love of the game by many players slightly less skilled than the major leaguers. If you count yourself in that legion of nonsalaried hitters, if all your swings are free—not just those on a 3-0 count—then read on and see how cross training can make you a better baseball player.

Physical Fitness Benefits of Baseball

As future Hall of Fame catcher Carlton Fisk once said, "Just playing baseball isn't enough to keep you in shape." (The chart on page 000 indicates this is fact.)

Potential Physical Fitness Benefits Provided by Baseball

Aerobic Capacity	2
Strength Upper Body	4
Strength Lower Body	3
Flexibility Upper Body	3
Flexibility Lower Body	3

These benefits assume the exerciser is following the principles of exercise as described in Chapter 3. Naturally there are some people who will gain more or less than the estimated benefit listed here.

4 = excellent	3 = good	2= fair	1 = minimal

When you are on the field you are standing still most of the time. With the exception of the relief pitchers and the on-deck batters, the other players spend the game sitting and waiting. Baseball fans who wish to question the value of cross training for baseball players will point to Babe Ruth, Detroit Tiger pitcher Mickey Lolich, and Tiger home-run champ Cecil Fielder as examples of outstanding players with less than outstanding physiques. Why, then, do baseball players need cross training?

It helps to be familiar with the physiological fact that additional body weight carried in the form of fat tissue does not contribute to power in throwing or hitting. Unnecessary fat tissue will slow a player down as he or she fields or runs the bases. Other benefits of fitness for baseball players are fewer injuries, faster recoveries from injuries, and longer careers.

To be fair, it must be noted that at every level, from Little League to the major leagues, that the great majority of today's baseball players are fit. Those players with all-round physical fitness achieve this status through serious cross-training conditioning performed in pre-season, after games, and during the off-season.

Carlton Fisk is one of the best-known examples of successful cross training for baseball. During the 1984–1985 off-season Fisk cross trained with weight lifting and then found it necessary to train during the season as well, even going so far as to keep the Chicago White Sox equipment manager in the weight room spotting Fisk for an hour *after* games. Fisk went on to enjoy a terrific season and batted in over a hundred runs.

Cross Training Prescription for Baseball

The ideal baseball player can run fast, throw hard and straight, catch well, hit often, and hit for power. Can you be a great baseball player without all of these skills? Absolutely. But if you wish to be the best baseball player you can be, you should develop your physical fitness potential in a way that complements the required skills of baseball.

Activities that can be performed for twenty minutes or

longer such as swimming, cycling, stair stepping, and aerobic dance will utilize many calories and help keep body fat low.

Cross Training for Baseball Strength

Three-time NCAA champion coach Jerry Kindall of the University of Arizona says strength is needed for good hitting:

> To be a good hitter, you must have a measure of physical strength. I have never seen a good hitter at the advanced levels of baseball who was weak and anemic. To accelerate a bat from a resting position to a speed that will literally overpower the pitched ball in the short distance of the swing requires a great amount of hands-wrist-forearm and upper body strength. **Weight training programs, which more and more are strengthening players in every sport,** are the chief factor behind the general surge of home runs and extra base hits these days in baseball.

To develop the muscle groups engaged in swinging a bat the exercises listed below are recommended. Except for wrist curls and tennis ball squeeze, you should do eight to twelve repetitions of each exercise. The weight should be set so that you can complete eight repetitions but not thirteen; that is, you reach muscular exhaustion *before* the thirteenth repetition. This system of performing at least eight repetitions but no more than twelve has repeatedly been found to be the most efficient method of training to increase strength.

Check with your coach before you begin your strength training program to be sure you are performing the exercises correctly.

Strength Training to Improve Hitting

Exercise	Muscle Groups	Reps	Workouts per Week
	Back Region		
Lower back machine	Erector spinae, quadratus lumborum	8–12	3
Lat pulldowns	Lattisimus dorsi	8–12	3
Seated rowing	Lattisimus dorsi, rear deltoids	8–12	3
	Shoulder Region		
Military press	Deltoids	8–12	3
Shrugs	Trapezius	8–12	3
Upright rowing	Lattisumus dorsi,	8–12	3
Lateral raises	Lateral deltoids	8–12	3
Forward raises	Anterior deltoids	8–12	3
Dips	Deltoids, triceps	8–12	3
	Arms		
Triceps pushdowns	Triceps	8–12	3
Curls	Biceps	8–12	3
Reverse curls	Biceps, radialis	8–12	3
Wrist curls	Radialis, ulnaris	To exhaustion	3
Tennis ball squeeze	Radialis, ulnaris, numerous hand muscles	To exhaustion	3

Improving Throwing

A heavy rope weighs three to five pounds, and jumping rope is recommended as an exercise for improving throwing. Begin with five sets of one minute each and work your way up to ten minutes without stopping, three times per week.

Cross Training for Speed in Baseball

The game of baseball requires sprinting. The distance involved most often is the sprint from home plate to first base, a distance of 90 feet. When you hit the ball past the outfielders you may have to sprint to second base (180 feet), third base (270 feet), or all around the bases back to home plate (360 feet). This last run is known as an inside-the-park home run because the ball doesn't go over the outfield wall. Outfielders run distances ranging from five feet to 120 feet, according to where the ball is hit.

The sprint to first after you hit a ground ball is very close to a pure sprint. You can run all out without looking at the ball or worrying about overrunning first base, as long as you run directly past first. If you veer into the base path between first and second base you are considered to be live in the base path and can be tagged out.

Running to other bases requires an awareness of the location of the ball and the fielder's handling of the ball. This knowledge is gained in a split-second glance toward the fielder, followed immediately by your decision— continue to the next base or stay where you are? The third base coach is supposed to help you with the decision.

Given these sprinting demands, what should baseball players do to cross train for speed?

Even before we discuss cross training for speed the matter of attitude must be addressed. You must bring the right attitude to every workout, every practice, and every game. When Tony LaRussa, manager of the Oakland Athletics, was asked why the A's were so pleased to obtain Ruben Sierra from the Texas Rangers in exchange for Oakland superstar outfielder Jose Canseco, LaRussa said about Sierra, "He is ready to do what it takes to win." This attitude relates to sprinting in baseball. If you want to be the best player you can be, you will *sprint* to first base on *every* ground ball just the way 3,000-hit third baseman George Brett does. Every once in a while an infielder will bobble an apparently easy play and you, the hustling player with the winning attitude, will cross first base before the infielder regains control of the ball. If you end up scoring and your team wins by one run your winning attitude made the difference. (The player with the poor attitude gives up once he or she sees the ball is hit directly to an infielder. Even if the infielder misplays the ball slightly this lackadaisical player is still thrown out.)

Is there a prescription for developing a winning attitude? Yes. You can develop a positive mindset while doing your sprint training. Before each sprint say to yourself "Hit the ball, sprint to first." In time the sprint to first becomes a reflex that follows the hit. After this attitude and maximum-effort sprint reflex are ingrained, you then begin developing judgment on line drive hits and other balls hit in the air so you will know whether or not you should be trying for second or third.

The maximum-effort reflex applies to outfielders, too. When the ball is hit in the air in your general direction you must be at *full speed* within a matter of steps and be thinking to yourself, "I can get to this ball." If you make the catch for the out, great, if not, you are quickly on top of the ball, fielding it and throwing it to the cutoff man.

Sprint Workout

On a track or running area, measure 90, 180, 270, and 360 feet. In yards you would measure 30, 60, 90, and 120—a lined football field would be convenient.

Wear running shoes and clothing. Jog easy for twelve to fifteen minutes. Stretch your hamstrings, quadriceps, achilles tendons, and lower back (see chapter 4 for stretching technique).

You will be doing a series of sprints at the four distances measured, but before you begin note that your first sprint after your warm-up should be done at no more than 80 percent of maximum intensity. You will gradually work your way to an all-out effort.

Sprint for the Cycle

Jog easy for 12 to 15 minutes. Then stretch your hamstrings, quadriceps, achilles tendons, and lower back.

FIRST SET

Distance	Intensity	Recovery
30 yards	80%	Jog back to start
60 yards	80%	Jog back to start
90 yards	80%	Jog back to start
120 yards	80%	Jog back to start

SECOND SET

Distance	Intensity	Recovery
30 yards	90%	Jog back to start
60 yards	90%	Jog back to start
90 yards	90%	Jog back to start
120 yards	90%	Jog back to start

THIRD SET

Distance	Intensity	Recovery
30 yards	100%	Walk back to start
60 yards	100%	Walk back to start
90 yards	100%	Walk back to start
120 yards	100%	Walk back to start

Do the fourth and fifth set the same as the third: 100% effort.

Cooldown: Jog slowly for two minutes. Walk slowly for two minutes. Repeat stretching exercises. Drink fluids as needed.

Cross Training for Baseball Quickness and Reflexes

In sport the difference between speed and quickness may be thought of in terms of the distance involved. Quickness can be defined as the ability to move up to ten feet rapidly. Examples of quickness in baseball abound. Infielders moving to catch a ball hit hard in their direction, outfielders making the quick run needed to snare the ball hit in front of them, the runner on first diving back to the bag to avoid being picked off.

Reflexes can be defined, in the context of sport, as those instantaneous movements performed in response to your opponent or an object of the game such as a ball. (The dictionary definition for physiological reflex is "a movement performed involuntarily." This definition does not match the sporting world's definition of *reflexes* which is voluntary movement.) Gold Glove winner Graig Nettles demonstrated great reflexes as a third baseman by snaring line drives hit by Hall of Fame catcher Johnny Bench when the Yankees met the Reds in the World Series.

The hitter with great reflexes can wait longer before beginning to swing. By waiting longer the hitter is able to see what type of pitch is coming and where the ball is headed. This "longer" wait consists of only a fraction of a second. Hitting a pitched baseball has been described as the single most difficult skill in sport. To improve the reflexes needed for hitting there is no better practice than batting practice itself.

The reflexes of the infielder can be cultivated, however, through such baseball drills as Pepper and hours of plain old fielding practice. There are several major league baseball players who got to the major leagues primarily because of hitting ability, but who then worked day in and day out on fielding reflexes until they became proficient. Hall of Fame third baseman Mike Shannon is an excellent example of such a player. Dedicated practice took Shannon from a liability at third to Gold Glove winner.

Cross-training activities that utilize gross motor movements similar to those performed in baseball are basketball, handball, racquetball, paddleball, and squash. Each of these sports calls for reactions and muscular flexibility comparable to those of infielders responding to a sharply hit ball. Full-court basketball includes the sprints discussed earlier since courts are 94 feet long. Playing any of these five sports three to five times per week during the off-season will allow you to regain your baseball fielding reflexes more rapidly when spring training begins.

Cross Training Recommendations for Baseball Players to Improve Overall Physical Fitness

The sport of baseball in and of itself does little to promote physical fitness for its participants, but baseball players have a large selection of cross-training activities from which to choose that do. All activities that stimulate the cardiovascular system are worthwhile choices for cross-training baseball players. Following is an outline for a cross-training program for a baseball player:

Baseball Cross-Training Program

Fitness Component	Activity	Frequency		
		Pre-Season	In-Season	Off-Season
Aerobic capacity	Basketball or racquet sports, other activities that meet principles of intensity, frequency, and duration	1x/week*	As needed	3x/week
Strength	Strength training	3x/week*	As needed	3x/week
Speed	Do "Sprint for the Cycle"	1–2x/week	As needed	1x/week
Quickness	Play similarly demanding sports	No	No	3x/week
Flexibility	Do flexibility training	3x/week	As needed	3x/week

*If you are on a team, follow your coach's instructions.

Cross Training for Basketball

At all levels, from grade schoolers shooting toward an eight-foot basket to college intramural gym rats, basketball is a fantastic game. Children begin dribbling as early as age three, and the sixty-two-year old governor of New York, Mario Cuomo, stays in shape by playing a tough brand of half-court basketball several times a week. In

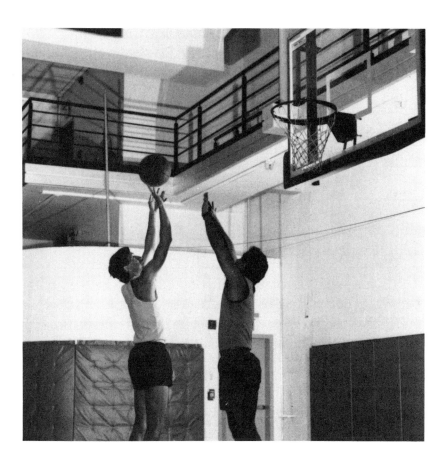

Cross training for basketball will help you improve your shooting and your defense.

fact, basketball is played and watched more than any other team game in the world.

In 1891 Dr. James Naismith invented basketball as a game that could be played indoors to fill the months between fall football and spring baseball. One hundred and one years after the first peach baskets were hung in a Springfield, Massachusetts, YMCA, the United States "Dream Team" showed the world the best American basketball players at the 1992 Olympics. By all accounts the dream team put on an awesome display of power and skill as the eleven NBA professionals and one collegian thoroughly dominated their Olympic opponents in Barcelona, Spain, en route to the gold medal.

Potential Physical Fitness
Benefits Provided by Basketball
▪ ▪

Aerobic Capacity	4
Strength Upper Body	3
Strength Lower Body	4
Flexibility Upper Body	3
Flexibility Lower Body	3

These benefits assume the exerciser is following the principles of exercise as described in Chapter 3. Naturally there are some people who will gain more or less than the estimated benefit listed here.

4 = excellent   3 = good   2 = fair   1 = minimal

Cross Training to Improve Basketball Performance

As you read earlier, Magic Johnson had great success with cross training for basketball in the fall of 1991. New York Knick center Patrick Ewing is another NBA superstar who cross trains, with weight lifting. Utah Jazz power forward deluxe, Karl Malone, cross trains by doing sprint repeats of Olympic intensity during the off-season and is known for his ability to run the floor on the fast break. His photograph in *Sports Illustrated* was accompanied by the caption, "Working with weights has helped Malone lift his level of play." Another NBA star known for cross training to improve performance is the Detroit Pistons rebounding/defensive specialist Dennis Rodman.

Cross Training for Basketball Strength

When playing defense it is your responsibility to fight past picks so you can stay close to the player you are guarding. There are also collisions on a basketball court, and the stronger you are the better you will survive them. When you and your opponent grab a loose ball at the same time, who will end up with control of the ball? If you are a guard, you can get caught in a switch and find yourself responsible for boxing out a bigger, stronger player. You need strength to do these things on the court.

Before the 1992–1993 NBA season began, New Jersey Nets coach Chuck Daly told 165-pound point guard Kenny Anderson he needed to "bulk up" in order to become one of the top point guards in the NBA. What Coach Daly really wanted was to have Kenny Anderson increase his muscle mass and strength so he would be able to withstand the pounding of an eighty-two-game season.

Whether you are a point guard, a point forward, or the biggest player in your league you will be more effective at your position if you cross train for basketball strength.

(*Safety Note:* Adolescents should review the program presented here with a coach or sports medicine professional to be sure their bodies are physically ready for strength training.)

Cross Training for Basketball Speed

Regarding your warm-up—if you are doing speed work immediately after a vigorous practice your muscles should already be warm and ready for high-intensity conditioning. If you have not just finished practice and your muscles are not ready for speed work you should do a proper warm-up.

Basketball speed calls for sprints of five to thirty yards. Front court players on a typical high school court will run twenty to twenty-five yards when filling a lane on a fast break, or when getting back on defense.

For years coaches have had players train for speed at the end of practice, even though the players do a lot of running during practice. This after-practice running is known by different names such as line drills, killers, suicides, or wind sprints. Whatever the name, the conditioning involved is usually some variation of the workout, which is described for you here.

Off-Season Basketball Training Program

Exercise	Primary Muscle Groups	Reps	Sets/Week
UPPER BODY			
Bench Press	Pectoralis major, anterior deltoids, triceps	8–12	3
Military Press	Deltoids, triceps	8–12	3
Triceps Presses	Triceps	8–12	3
Pushups	Pectoralis major, triceps	To exhaustion	2
Dips	Triceps, anterior deltoids, pectoralis major	To exhaustion	2
Reverse Curls	Biceps brachii, brachoradialis	To exhaustion	2
LOWER BODY			
Double Leg Press	Quadriceps, gluteus maximus	8–12	3
Leg Extension	Quadriceps	8–12	3
Leg Flexion	Hamstrings	8–12	3
ABDOMINAL AREA			

Refer to page 63 in chapter 5. Be sure to do your abdominal work because strong abdominals are valuable for maintaining proper defensive position, absorbing flying elbows, and hanging tough in the fourth quarter.

Fill the Lane & Get Back on Defense: A Basketball Speed Workout

Warm-up (if necessary): Jog easy for twelve to fifteen minutes. Then stretch your hamstrings, quadriceps, achilles tendons, and lower back.

On the Court

Running the Lines: Line up on the baseline.

Get yourself mentally prepared for a 100% effort.
At your own signal you will start.
Run to near foul line, touch floor
run back to baseline, touch floor (= 1 line),
run to half-court, touch, run to baseline, touch (= 2 lines),
run to far foul line, touch, run to baseline, touch (= 3 lines),
run to opposite baseline, touch, run to orig. baseline (= 4 lines).

Touching the floor at each line makes you bend your knees and lower your center of gravity. For basketball quickness, lower is better.

Running the lines in the manner described here equals running the court four times without any break in the action.

If you give a maximum effort you will realize right away why running the lines is called things like "killers" and "suicides." It may help you endure the pain if you remind yourself that such effort is necessary if you wish to reach your full potential as an athlete.

If you have a teammate or friend who can time you on your first effort you can use that time as a goal for subsequent efforts.

Line Drill Workouts

Level I
Run 4 lines, rest 3:00, run 4 lines, rest 3:00, run 2 lines, rest 3:00, 2 lines, rest, stretch.

Level II
4 lines 4x, rest 2:30 between
2 lines 4x, rest 1:15 between, stretch

Level III
4 lines 6x, rest 2:00 between, stretch

> **Level IV**
> 4 lines 8x, rest 1:30 between, stretch
>
> **Level V**
> 4 lines 10x, rest 1:00 between, stretch
>
> A useful variation of the line drills involves running forward to the line in front of you and backpedaling to the baseline. This is a movement performed when getting back on defense. Backpedaling develops balance as well.

Cross Training for Basketball Quickness

• *Patter Drill.* Begin in a defensive stance with your knees bent, back fairly straight, feet slightly wider than shoulder width, palms facing up. On your own start signal you "patter" with your feet by picking up one foot at a time about two inches off the ground, then repeating this movement as fast as you possibly can. Your heels should not touch the ground at any time while you are doing the Patter Drill. If you are working hard your quadriceps will hurt by the end of each set.

• *Ski Drill.* Begin in a modified defensive stance; that is, knees bent, head up, but legs together and hands held as you would for jogging. On your own start signal you jump with both feet *to the side*, over any line (or imaginary line) on the court. You jump just high enough to get both feet off the ground and over to the other side of the line. Then you jump back to your starting position, and so forth.

• *Single-Leg Ski Drill.* Jump from side to side just like the regular ski drill but on one leg.

• *Box Drills.* Begin in a modified defensive stance (as in Ski Drill above). Look down at the floor and imagine you can see a box twelve inches square; place your feet on the lower left-hand corner of the box. On your own start signal you will jump with both feet straight ahead to the top left-hand corner of the box, then across to the top right-hand corner, then backward to the lower right-hand corner, and finally back to your starting position.

• *Defensive Sliding.* Begin in a defensive stance with feet straddling one of the foul lanes. On your own start signal slide one foot at a time across the foul lane toward the other side of the foul lane. Once your outside foot passes the other lane line you immediately change directions and slide back across the three-second lane to your starting point. You slide back and forth as fast as you can. *Note:* Stay down in a good defensive position and be sure your feet do not get closer than twelve inches apart at any time.

• *Jumping Rope.* Jumping rope is explained in chapter 11. It is an excellent cross-training option for basketball quickness because it requires rapid, continuous footwork and forearm muscular endurance.

Pre-Season Training

Pre-season basketball practice is supposed to be physically demanding. You will have to see how much energy you have left after practice to put into cross training. If you are competing at the high school or collegiate level you must factor in time for studying. If, along with company team pre-season basketball practices, you are working full-time and/or are responsible for children you will evaluate your available time for cross training accordingly. For many players the goal of three to six workouts per week is appropriate. If the team only meets once per week you need at least two cross-training workouts in addition.

Serious college players and professionals will do strength training after practice during the pre-season, but if that's more than you need don't worry about it. Recovering between workouts is very important in order to have a successful, injury-free season.

Cross Training and Boxing

Boxing is also known as pugilism and prizefighting. "Pugilism" derives from the Greek *pugme*, a fist or fight with fists, and the Latin *pugnus*, fist, and *pugil*, boxer. The first evidence of boxing as a sport is found in Egyptian hieroglyphics believed to date from 4000 B.C. Boxing accompanied the spread of civilization from Egypt to Mesopotamia, Crete, Greece, and Rome. Centuries later it came to England, and then to the United States.

Boxers have been cross training for many years. Sparring is another word for boxing, but it is often used to refer to boxing done in the ring for purposes of learning and practice—as opposed to tournament boxing, which is performed in front of judges, referees, and spectators. Sparring is an extremely demanding activity during which the athlete's body is subjected to a high level of physical punishment and exhaustion. Due to the physical abuse of boxing's learning sessions, a boxer's practice time in the ring is limited. Cross training allows boxers to condition their bodies without being pummeled by a practice partner.

Boxers cross train by doing "roadwork" (jogging), abdominal work (very high repetitions), strength training, jumping rope, and chasing chickens (that is, if you wish to train like the movie boxer Rocky Balboa). Four of these five methods of training are discussed in *Cross Training*.

The former heavyweight champion of the world, Evander Holyfield, is widely acknowledged to have used cross training in the most scientific manner of any boxer in history. Through his training Holyfield built his body from lightweight stature into a bona fide heavyweight physique. When he was in his prime, he was always superbly conditioned and had a reputation of getting stronger as his fights moved into the later rounds.

Today many people find the boxing cross-training workout and atmosphere so beneficial that they are signing up to train in boxing gyms even though they don't plan on getting in the ring.

If you decide to do boxing cross training you will enjoy an excellent degree of all-round physical fitness. The only component of fitness boxing cross training does not address directly is lower body flexibility. You can do the stretches presented in chapter 4 to remedy this.

Potential Physical Fitness Benefits Provided by Boxing

Aerobic Capacity	4
Strength Upper Body	4
Strength Lower Body	4
Flexibility Upper Body	4
Flexibility Lower Body	3

These benefits assume the exerciser is following the principles of exercise as described in Chapter 3. Naturally there are some people who will gain more or less than the estimated benefit listed here.

4 = excellent	3 = good	2 = fair	1 = minimal

Should you decide to learn the techniques involved in the "sweet science," be sure to take lessons—and don't forget to duck.

Cross Training for Bowling

Bowling pins and a bowling ball, both made of stone, were found in an Egyptian tomb dating back to 5200 B.C. Polynesians of ancient times rolled stones at objects sixty feet away, the exact distance from the foul line to the head pin in today's game.

Most of the 60 million American recreational bowlers trying to roll a perfect game throughout the year enjoy the social atmosphere of the bowling alley. It's easy to visit with your friends between turns. You can have all kinds of refreshments and keep track of a game or some other event on television. Then, when it's your turn, you shift into your concentration mode for a minute or two (less if you throw a strike) and then you can relax again for a while.

There is not a great deal of movement involved in bowling—only three, four, or five steps per approach, knees bend, and one shoulder rotates—so physiologists rate the activity of bowling as providing relatively little in the way of real physical fitness benefits (see Appendix A). Bowlers have much to gain by cross training with a simple three days per week exercise program.

Potential Physical Fitness Benefits Provided by Bowling

Aerobic Capacity	1
Strength Upper Body	2
Strength Lower Body	1
Flexibility Upper Body	3
Flexibility Lower Body	2

These benefits assume the exerciser is following the principles of exercise as described in Chapter 3. Naturally there are some people who will gain more or less than the estimated benefit listed here.

4 = excellent   3 = good   2 = fair   1 = minimal

Here are a few ideas for incorporating cross training into your bowling outings.

Could three members of your bowling foursome walk (or jog) to the alley and the fourth take the car so everyone could have a ride home at the end of the night? What about riding a bicycle to the bowling alley? Or learning how to maneuver on in-line skates?

To improve your flexibility while out bowling you can do a number of stretches between turns as described in Chapter 4.

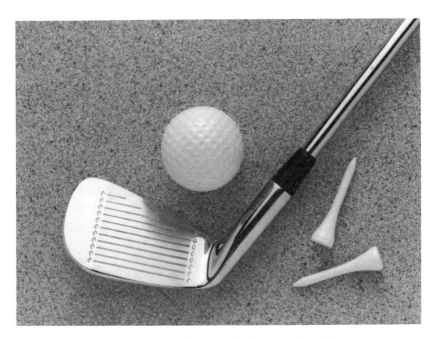

Golfers have much to gain by cross training.

Cross Training for Golf

No one has ever played a perfect game of golf. The legendary Ben Hogan once said he rarely hit more than five good shots in a round. Perhaps the best aspect of the sport is the opportunity it offers for continuing improvement. No sport goes beyond golf in its demand for precise motor control of large muscle groups combined with laser-quality focus on the task. Since you can play golf well without possessing a sprinter's speed or a power lifter's strength, people of all ages can strive for and achieve better swings and lower scores on their favorite courses, year after year after year.

Two of the first American golfers with recognized cross-training ability were "Babe" Didrikson Zaharias (discussed in chapter 1 as the greatest all-round female athlete of the first half of the twentieth century), and the enduring Sam Snead. In his youth Snead played tackle football, tournament tennis, and ran the hundred yard dash in ten seconds. But, he says, "Golf was the game that captured my imagination and my life."

Do golfers need cross training? In their book *Golf Today* St. Paul, MN: West Publishing, 1989), professional golfer J. C. Snead and Professor John Johnson state:

> The average golfer works with an inefficient body, neither as strong nor as flexible as it needs to be for an adequate performance. Yet, everyone can increase flexibility and strength. For the average golfer who has not done flexibility or strength exercises before, the improvement is drastic once such exercises are begun. For the well-conditioned athlete, improvement is slower but it is nevertheless inevitable. Players at every level will benefit from (the right) exercises.

Cross Training for Golf Flexibility

• *Abdominal Twist.* Face away from a wall with your feet slightly farther apart than shoulder width. Slowly, turn toward the wall until you can place both hands on the wall at about chest level. Hold this position for ten to thirty seconds. Repeat to the opposite side and do four more sets of turns in each direction.

• *Triceps Stretch.* From a standing position, raise one arm in front of your body until it is parallel to the ground. Keeping the arm fairly straight and parallel to the ground, rotate it at the shoulder and bring it in toward your chest. Now place your other hand under your triceps (near your elbow) and pull your arm gently toward your body. Hold for ten to thirty seconds. Repeat to the opposite side and do four more sets in each direction.

• To learn how to do other stretches helpful to golfers see chapter 4 and do: groin stretch and the lateral trunk stretch.

Cross Training for Golf Strength

• Abdominal obliques (see chapter 5).
• Wrist curls and triceps extensions (see Cross Training for Baseball, page 101).

Potential Physical Fitness Benefits Provided by Golf

Aerobic Capacity	2
Strength Upper Body	3
Strength Lower Body	1
Flexibility Upper Body	4
Flexibility Lower Body	2

These benefits assume the exerciser is following the principles of exercise as described in Chapter 3. Naturally there are some people who will gain more or less than the estimated benefit listed here.

4 = excellent   3 = good   2 = fair   1 = minimal

Golf and Physical Fitness

All-pro linebacker Lawrence Taylor of the New York Giants was once asked if playing golf is a good way to work out. He is reported to have answered "Yes, if you are carrying your clubs over your shoulder as you walk the course." With the typical golf club bag weighing in at thirty pounds, and the average eighteen-hole golf course requiring four to five miles of walking, only a small number of golfers can be found following this suggestion.

If you are prepared to add the flexibility and strength-training exercises, then the missing components for complete physical fitness as elevated here would be aerobic capacity and muscular endurance. To improve your aerobic fitness you should cross train by doing one of the aerobic activities described in chapter 11, or if you have the time and inclination, join a team and play a sport that offers aerobic training through its practices and games.

Whichever aerobic option you select remember to do three workouts per week, twenty to thirty minutes at a time, and get your heart rate into your target zone.

Of course, when you do get to the golf course, you should always try to walk the course. (Unfortunately, some courses now require that you rent a golf cart.)

Cross Training for the Martial Arts

All sportsmen should do cross training. Martial arts are way behind in this area.

—Joe Lewis,
former world full-contact karate champion

The word *martial* comes from Mars, the Roman god of war and agriculture. The term "martial arts" has come to refer to both a philosophy of life and various forms of one-on-one combat. In his *Dictionary of the Martial Arts* (Rutland, VT: Tuttle, 1991), Louis Frederic lists thirty-nine forms of martial arts, from aikido to yamato-ryu. Hundreds of techniques are involved in these different forms.

In the United States judo and karate are the best known and most widely practiced forms of the martial arts. By reading about cross training for judo and karate, practitioners of others forms will be able to compare their disciplines, evaluate their needs, and incorporate cross training accordingly.

Many people begin judo or karate classes to achieve a sense of empowerment. If they stay with their classes for any reasonable period of time they learn the rules, etiquette, and philosophy that are integral to these sports.

Cross Training for Judo

The philosophy of judo was formulated in the 1880s by a Japanese educator named Jigaro Kano. From various ancient combat arts, he synthesized two new forms, one for physical education and the other for self-defense. Kano believed that if the student would obey his *sensei* (teacher), observe the strict rules of etiquette, and train hard, he

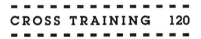

would learn self-control and become humble, resolute, and judicious, traits that would give him an advantage over other people.

Potential Physical Fitness Benefits Provided by Judo

Aerobic Capacity	2
Strength Upper Body	4
Strength Lower Body	4
Flexibility Upper Body	4
Flexibility Lower Body	4

These benefits assume the exerciser is following the principles of exercise as described in Chapter 3. Naturally there are some people who will gain more or less than the estimated benefit listed here.

4 = excellent   3 = good   2 = fair   1 = minimal

Today the principal physical techniques of judo are throwing and grappling. This chart displays the potential physical fitness benefits of judo, which provides balanced fitness in all areas with the possible exception of aerobic capacity. If your sensei includes the proper amount of running as part of the class you may already be aerobically fit. If there is no running, or too little, then your cross-training workouts for judo should involve activities that provide aerobic fitness. You can cross train by doing any of the other aerobic activities described in this book three times per week for twenty minutes at least per workout with your heart rate in your target zone.

If you wish to cross train for the purpose of augmenting your competitive performance in judo you should consider the following workouts:

Strength training for judo: Follow the overall body workout described in chapter 5.

Quickness training for judo: Boxing and wrestling will enhance quickness and add to your muscular endurance at the same time. Jumping rope is an excellent cross-training activity for judo because it demands rapid footwork. Once you have mastered the basics of jumping rope, try double jumps (chapter 11). You will spin the rope around you twice per jump. Double jumps make you work anaerobically and therefore will help your sparring stamina.

Cross Training for Karate

Karate enjoys greater fame than judo throughout the general public in the United States, probably due in part to the spectacular movies of martial arts champion Bruce Lee. Yet karate is actually a generic term for a group of Asian fighting methods in which hand and foot blows are the principal techniques.

Accounts of the origin of karate vary, but there is fairly general agreement that it derives from a form of hand-to-hand combat that originated in India and later was introduced to China by a Buddhist monk. In the early 1900s, Funakoshi Gichin, an Okinawan and the founder of modern karate, introduced karate to Japan in a series of lectures and demonstrations. The Japanese ideogram that represents the word karate can be translated as "empty" (kara) "hand" (te) or as "Chinese" (kara) "hand" (te).

As with judo, men, women, and children practice karate for self-defense, competition, and exercise. Although the techniques between the two sports are quite different, karate is similar to judo when it comes to potential physical fitness benefits.

Potential Physical Fitness Benefits Provided by Karate

Aerobic Capacity	2
Strength Upper Body	3
Strength Lower Body	4
Flexibility Upper Body	4
Flexibility Lower Body	4

These benefits assume the exerciser is following the principles of exercise as described in Chapter 3. Naturally there are some people who will gain more or less than the estimated benefit listed here.

4 = excellent   3 = good   2 = fair   1 = minimal

For balanced physical fitness karate devotees should engage in an activity that develops aerobic endurance. Jumping rope is an excellent option because it provides aerobic endurance, requires quick feet, and develops muscular endurance in the wrists and forearms. With improved overall fitness you will be able to train longer in each practice session. To attain greater anaerobic capabilities try the double-jump workout (chapter 11).

World kickboxing champion Kathy Long builds aerobic endurance by running up (and walking down) stadium stairs. She also does wind sprints (see the basketball speed workout in this chapter for a sprint workout you can do. If you don't have access to a gym, use the lines on an outdoor basketball court.)

Strength training for karate: Follow the overall muscular development workout recommendations described in chapter 5.

Reverse Cross-Training: Using Martial Arts to Improve Performance in Other Sports

No less a superstar than the National Basketball Association's all-time leading scorer, Kareem Abdul-Jabbar, has used martial arts during his basketball career. "It [martial arts and yoga stretching] definitely enabled me to prolong my basketball career," says Abdul-Jabbar. On the question of why professional athletes are turning to martial arts as a supplement to their training, Abdul-Jabbar states, "I think it has to do with the whole idea of a total package of conditioning in the mental warrior aspect, which is something you have to understand in a competitive sport."

Martial arts maneuvers and training methods have a lot to offer athletes involved in other sports as well. Karate black belt Greg Silva stresses movements in his Florida karate classes that develop the body parts necessary for soccer and baseball skills. As Silva's younger students develop these moves in training, their soccer and baseball performances improve.

Cross Training for Racquet Sports

The six great racquet sports have a great deal in common. The aerobic and anaerobic physiological demands on the body for playing these sports are more alike than not. You can be on the court for hours (aerobic conditioning) and have to move short distances quickly again and again (anaerobic conditioning). The motor control patterns and mental aspects are comparable as well. All six sports require hand-eye coordination and stroke mastery. Athletes in each sport are expected to have an ability to hone in on the ball to the exclusion of all other stimuli—going into the "zone" it is sometimes called.

The popularity of racquet sports can be attributed to

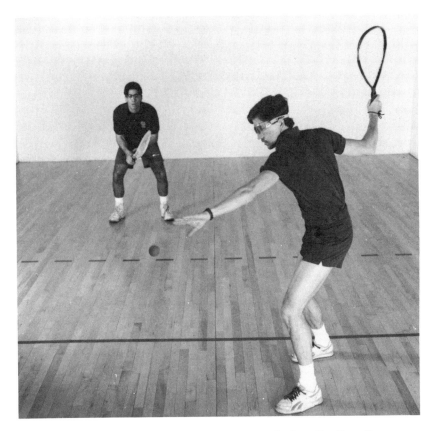

Racquetball is a wonderful cross training choice. It offers the challenge of a skill sport, competition, and excellent conditioning benefits.

several factors. At the amateur level, they are relatively inexpensive (with exceptions like advanced lessons or indoor court time); they are fast paced; when played vigorously they offer a wonderful aerobic workout and fairly good overall fitness; and they are all fun to play whether you are a beginner running around your backhand or a skilled athlete with a wicked serve.

Racquet Sport Beginnings

Sport	Date	Place
Handball	Ancient Rome	Rome
Squash	1840s	England
Badminton	1860s	India
Tennis	1873	England
Paddleball	1930s	United States
Racquetball	1940s	United States

Potential Physical Fitness Benefits Provided by Badminton

Aerobic Capacity	3
Strength Upper Body	2
Strength Lower Body	3
Flexibility Upper Body	4
Flexibility Lower Body	3

These benefits assume the exerciser is following the principles of exercise as described in Chapter 3. Naturally there are some people who will gain more or less than the estimated benefit listed here.

4 = excellent   3 = good   2 = fair   1 = minimal

Potential Physical Fitness
Benefits Provided by Handball

Aerobic Capacity	4
Strength Upper Body	2
Strength Lower Body	3
Flexibility Upper Body	4
Flexibility Lower Body	3

These benefits assume the exerciser is following the principles of exercise as described in Chapter 3. Naturally there are some people who will gain more or less than the estimated benefit listed here.

4 = excellent   3 = good   2 = fair   1 = minimal

Potential Physical Fitness
Benefits Provided by Paddleball

Aerobic Capacity	4
Strength Upper Body	2
Strength Lower Body	3
Flexibility Upper Body	4
Flexibility Lower Body	4

These benefits assume the exerciser is following the principles of exercise as described in Chapter 3. Naturally there are some people who will gain more or less than the estimated benefit listed here.

4 = excellent   3 = good   2 = fair   1 = minimal

Potential Physical Fitness
Benefits Provided by Racquetball

- -

Aerobic Capacity	4
Strength Upper Body	2
Strength Lower Body	3
Flexibility Upper Body	4
Flexibility Lower Body	3

These benefits assume the exerciser is following the principles of exercise as described in Chapter 3. Naturally there are some people who will gain more or less than the estimated benefits listed here.

4 = excellent   3 = good   2 = fair   1 = minimal

Potential Physical Fitness
Benefits Provided by Squash

- - - - - - - - - - - - - - - - - - -

Aerobic Capacity	4
Strength Upper Body	2
Strength Lower Body	3
Flexibility Upper Body	4
Flexibility Lower Body	3

These benefits assume the exerciser is following the principles of exercise as described in Chapter 3. Naturally there are some people who will gain more or less than the estimated benefit listed here.

4 = excellent   3 = good   2 = fair   1 = minimal

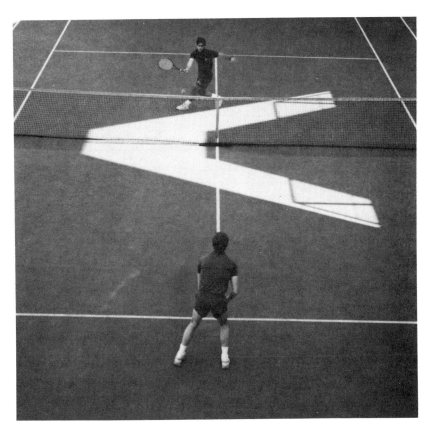

Singles tennis can provide outstanding overall physical fitness (see Appendix B).

Potential Physical Fitness
Benefits Provided by Tennis (Singles)

Aerobic Capacity	4	
Strength Upper Body	3	(for dominant arm)
Strength Lower Body	4	
Flexibility Upper Body	4	
Flexibility Lower Body	4	

These benefits assume the exerciser is following the principles of exercise as described in Chapter 3. Naturally there are some people who will gain more or less than the estimated benefit listed here.

4 = excellent   3 = good   2 = fair   1 = minimal

Potential Physical Fitness
Benefits Provided by Tennis (Doubles)

Aerobic Capacity	3
Strength Upper Body	3 (for dominant arm)
Strength Lower Body	3
Flexibility Upper Body	4
Flexibility Lower Body	3

These benefits assume the exerciser is following the principles of exercise as described in Chapter 3. Naturally there are some people who will gain more or less than the estimated benefit listed here.

4 = excellent   3 = good   2 = fair   1 = minimal

Cross Training for Racquet Sport Quickness

To be effective playing racquet sports you should have a quick mind, quick feet, and quick hand-eye reflexes. You must make quick decisions, position yourself quickly, and swing quickly. However, each racquet sport does differ when it comes to wrist action. The light badminton racquet can be handled with a whipping, slashing movement as you hit the floating shuttlecock, whereas the ground strokes of tennis call for quick racquet preparation and a firm wrist on contact with the ball. Therefore your cross training should be directed toward footwork quickness and conditioning. Later on you will incorporate drills to perfect your stroke.

Touching the Tentacles: The Octopus Drill

Warm-up: Jog slowly for five to ten minutes.

Stretching: Do the major muscle group stretches as described in chapter 4. Even though you will be swinging at imaginary objects, keep your flexibility routine intact and stretch the shoulder area, triceps, and wrists a second time.

Situate yourself in the middle of your playing area facing the net or front wall with racquet in hand.

1. On your own start signal (or by a partner's command) run straight ahead as quickly as you can to within one stride of the net or wall. Make a balanced stop, then take a perfect swing at an imaginary ball (or shuttlecock), then backpedal to your starting point.

2. Immediately run to the next "tentacle" in the top right corner of your court, do a balanced stop, take a perfect swing at an imaginary ball, run back to your starting point.

3. Work your way around the court until you have touched all eight tentacles.

By moving to the eight different spots on the court without having to watch a flying object, you can concentrate on your stride, your balance when you stop, and body mechanics when you swing. It's true you do all these movements when you are playing a game, but you tend to do them without being aware of whether you are doing them *well*. Doing this drill will help you develop a controlled running style so you can cover the court efficiently and quickly.

Do the Octopus Drill by tentacle touches or time. On the indoor courts you will probably have to go around twice (16 touches), or for one to three minutes, to get conditioning benefits. Then rest as needed up to two minutes and do it again. Do five sets, then do your stroke drills, and then play a game.

Cross Training for Racquet Sport Stamina

Stamina, or aerobic endurance, refers here to the ability to play your sport for an extended period of time, such as one hour or more without becoming fatigued to point that you were slower getting to the ball, or injured (for example, leg cramps).

It has been estimated that three sets of singles tennis can require running the equivalent of five miles. It is safe to say that an athlete playing any of the racquet sports for forty-five minutes continuously would run the equivalent of two to three miles. However, many racquet sport players can only make the necessary court and partner arrangements for one match per week. One squash challenge per week will not keep you in shape to play your best, so you should cross train by running twice a week, two to three miles at a time. If you have the body, the attitude, and the time you can run longer. You can do interval training once a week, too, to further enhance your cardiovascular capabilities. (See Cross Training for Basketball in this chapter for a sample interval training workout that can be applied to racquet sport conditioning.)

You can cross train for racquet sport stamina by doing other activities besides running. Chapter 11 offers options that provide excellent aerobic endurance benefits and are fun to learn as well. Whatever your choice, remember the principles of exercise (chapter 3): Intensity—heart rate should be in your target zone. Frequency—three or more workouts per week. Duration—twenty to sixty minutes per week.

Cross Training for Strength in the Stroke Sports

Your stroke technique is critical for adroit performance. To master strokes you must practice carefully and precisely. But what if you hit the ball properly and lose the point because you hit it too weakly? In other words, your opponent gets to a ball that should have been a winner for you and blasts it back past you. If you need more power you should be cross training for strength by lifting weights.

The muscle groups you will need to train are the abdominals, forearms, triceps, and deltoids. When you increase strength of any given muscle group you can normally expect to experience improvement in that muscle group's endurance as well. Thus the tried and tested 8–12 repetition method of strength training will be effective for you. Remember you must set the weights so that you can reach muscular exhaustion at some point between 8 and 12 repetitions. When you can complete 12 reps you are ready for an increase in weight, and you may lower the reps back to 8.

If you have the time, you should consider applying the concept of specificity (explained in chapter 3) to this part of your cross-training program. You should do a second set at a lower weight. Set the weight so that you are able to do at least 24 repetitions but not more than 36. In this manner you will be stimulating the demands of the stroke sports— repeated muscular contradictions.

To learn the exact exercises that will strengthen the aforementioned muscle groups, and for more information on muscular development, refer to chapter 5.

Cross Training for Racquet Sport Flexibility

Basic cross training for racquet sport flexibility is known to many athletes but generally underutilized. Follow these workout recommendations for flexibility and you may expect one or more of the following benefits:

1. An ability to extend and handle shots you could not reach before.
2. Reduced risk of muscle pull, tendon strain, and other injuries.
3. Less stiffness the morning after a tough match.

The Workout

- Jog 5 minutes slowly.
- Hit lightly for 5 minutes.
- Stop playing and stretch all major muscle groups once; then stretch shoulder, triceps, and wrist a second time.
- Play your games.
- When you are done playing, stretch again.

Get it into your mind that the stretching done when you are finished playing is part of your workout.

Cross Training for the Racquet Sports by Season

While it is possible to play your sport year-round, few athletes are able to maintain true peak performances for twelve months straight. Some sports have clearly defined seasons and the athlete adjusts his or her training program accordingly. American football, for example, is in-season during the fall. Football players who participate in "spring football" are doing organized off-season training, but they do not have games against other schools. The football pre-season is roughly July and August.

Racquet sports, on the other hand (ambidextrously speaking?), do not have such a standardized season. Some racquet sport athletes play one game outdoors when the weather is mild and switch racquets for an indoor game in winter. Other racquet sport athletes don't like to tamper with their stroke and stay with their first love throughout the year.

If you take the time to think through your competitive goals (beat your friend more often?) and fitness needs (smaller love handles; that is, reduce body fat?), you will be able to devise an annual training plan for yourself. A plan will be extremely useful to you and to your family. Sit down with a note pad, a twelve-month calendar, and *Cross Training*. In a half-hour you will have developed your own annual cross-training plan.

Let's look at one example of a typical recreational

athlete who has been seasonally cross training for tennis the past eight years.

An associate professor of psychology at John Jay College, David Brandt is forty-nine years old and has been playing recreational tennis for twenty years. His greatest achievement in the tennis world? "Not my own play," he responded. "Teaching my daughter Karen to play tennis is my best accomplishment in the sport." Karen had a great tennis career at Hunter College, winning the singles championship in the City University of New York Tennis Tournament in 1988, 1989, and 1990.

"She followed my lead in terms of doing other activities, even though we didn't call our workouts cross training at the time. It's my feeling that by spending some time away from tennis Karen always returned to the court with an eagerness to practice that helped her game."

Since Dave doesn't compete in club or local tournaments he has two seasons but no pre-season. From May through September he is in-season and plays singles tennis twice a week. During those five months he supplements his tennis workouts with a stretching routine, four to six miles of running per week, upper body work with twenty-pound dumbbells, pushups, indoor and outdoor cycling.

Dave's "off-season" is really an indoor season because he continues to play tennis once a week and cross train even when it's too cold to play outside. From October to May Dave is an active member of the John Jay College Cardiovascular Fitness Center. His twice weekly cross-training workout consists of twenty minutes of aerobic exercise on either the cross-country ski machine, the Stairmaster, the treadmill, or the Lifecycle. For strength training he begins with the four Nautilus machines: the abdominal, the lower back, the multibiceps, and the triceps. He finishes his strength training with a set on the leg curl and the leg extension machines. Finally, he does his stretching.

Based on the Rating of Perceived Exertion Scale (explained in chapter 3), Dave does his workouts at a level of 13—Somewhat hard. He points out that because of his cross training he is able to play an hour and a half of singles tennis without getting tired.

Dave likes downhill skiing for the thrill it offers. He is a licensed pilot and loves the feeling of self-determination and solitude he experiences while soaring in the New England area. His next physical challenge? "I am thinking about a childhood dream—doing a trek to the Himalayas."

Cross Training for Swimmers

As the Physical Fitness Benefits table shows (see page 286), swimming provides wonderfully balanced physical fitness. So, if swimming is easy on your body and provides overall fitness, why do swimmers need to cross train? Surprisingly enough, there are several reasons swimmers benefit from cross training.

Potential Physical Fitness Benefits Provided by Swimming

Aerobic Capacity	4
Strength Upper Body	4
Strength Lower Body	3
Flexibility Upper Body	4
Flexibility Lower Body	3

These benefits assume the exerciser is following the principles of exercise as described in Chapter 3. Naturally there are some people who will gain more or less than the estimated benefit listed here.

4 = excellent	3 = good	2 = fair	1 = minimal

Swimmers need to cross train on terrain . . .

. . . if doing too many laps is causing any type of overuse injury
(the shoulder is the joint swimmers injure most often).

. . . if you are suffering from any type of respiratory illness
(when you have a mild cold, for example, a light workout on land is probably a better workout choice than getting in the water because you won't get chilled or spread germs).

. . . if you have any type of infection or rash
(swimmers are more prone to ear infections than other athletes).

. . . if the "black lines and bubbles" are getting to you
(you may be ready for the visual stimulation enjoyed during a scenic jog or bicycle outing).

. . . if you need a break from group workouts
(you love your masters team companions, but more space during your personal exercise time is what you would prefer for a few months).

. . . if your pool is unavailable for any length of time
(the pool is being repaired or you have to travel).

The story of thirty-two-year-old investment banker John Cashman is typical of swimmers who discover cross training.

Beginning at age six, John swam competitively for sixteen years. Even before he had finished his studies at Dartmouth he knew he was going to need a break from flip turns. Shortly after his last swim meet he began cross training by going for a short jog. "I was surprised at how sore my legs were after only a two-mile run, because I felt I was in excellent shape from all my swimming. But I was so happy to have another workout option that I knew I would stay with my early morning runs."

Weight lifting is another example of a cross-training activity popular with swimmers. United States 1992 Olympic swim coach Eddie Reese has always believed in the importance of weight lifting for his swimmers, and Dr. James Counsilman, U.S. Olympic swim coach in 1964 and 1976, said in 1988, "Swimmers of the past avoided building strength [through weight lifting]. Most of the swimmers of today use strength exercises in their programs." Coach Counsilman's observation is important for swimmers who wish to cross train to improve performance.

Cross Training to Improve Swim Performance

Your body and your swim goals are unique. If you have a swim coach be sure to discuss your interest in cross training with him or her before you begin cross training.

Better swimming means swimming faster, farther, more efficiently, or some combination of the three. The *first* element of better swimming is better stroke technique, and improved technique is developed through hours of drills and laps—in the pool. Next comes more demanding swim workouts—intervals and distance work. After you understand the relative importance of these first two elements of better swimming then you are ready to add cross training.

The table below is presented as an example of a six-week pre-season cross-training program for improving 50-meter freestyle sprint speed. If you are interested in improving your time for a different distance you will need to assess the physical demands of your event and adapt your cross training accordingly.

This cross-training program emphasizes strength development and overall physical conditioning. Strength training is done three to five days per week. If you feel the need to take a day off and let your muscles recover, do so. Your anaerobic capabilities will be enhanced through the interval training that uses the fast-twitch muscle fibers that supply the power in sprint swimming. Cycling and in-line skating are appropriate for sprint swim training because they help strengthen the hip and thigh muscles. Combining these activities with squats develops the overall lower body power needed for top performance in sprint swimming.

Any in-season cross-training program for swimming would shift the emphasis to actual swim workouts.

50-Meter Sprint 6-Week Cross-Training Program

Monday	Tuesday	Wednesday	Thursday	Friday	Saturday	Sunday
Warm-up	Warm-up	Warm-up	Repeat Monday	Repeat Tuesday	Repeat Wednesday	Rest
Abdominal workout	Abs	Swim bench speed workout				
Bench press	Seated rowing					
Overhead press	Front-lat pull-downs					
Squats	Curls					
Swim bench speed work	Triceps extensions					
	Cycling Intervals 45 min.	In-line Skating 30 min.		Running Intervals 50 to 100 yards		

NOTE: See chapter 5 for explanation of the different weight-lifting exercises, guidelines for setting the weight, and prescription for repetitions. Interval training is explained in chapter 3. For cycling information see page 210, for in-line skating see page 215, and for running refer to page 103.

Selecting Your Swimming Cross-Training Option

If you are getting out of the water to allow a shoulder or some other upper body part to heal, you can maintain your aerobic capacity by cross training with any of the following:

- Stair climbing machines
- Jogging—indoors or outdoors
- Aerobic dancing (avoid any arm movements that are uncomfortable)
- Step classes

Getting started and setting your workout prescription for these activities is explained in chapter 6.

If you need to stay dry while an ear infection heals or your cold clears up, you can cross train with just about any land activity described in this book.

If you are in need of a new view, choose your cross-

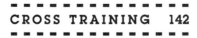

training option with scenery in mind. The beauty of nature can be seen in still life along the outdoor trail and in moving bodies indoors where other cross trainers hail.

If it's solitude you seek, you'll want to be self-sufficient. If you live alone you can set up indoor exercise equipment at home. You will find lots of ideas in the chapter 11 subsection, "Cross Training with Indoor Equipment." If you need to get away from your swim pals and get out of the house, jogging, outdoor cycling, and in-line skating are a few of your best options.

If your main concern is maintaining good upper body muscle tone while you are not swimming you should consider strength training, the *Gravitron* workout (chapter 5) and rock climbing (chapter 11).

If you would like to maintain both upper body muscle tone and aerobic capacity your best cross-training options are:

- Cross-country skiing
- Cross-country ski machine
- Rowing
- Rowing machine
- Upper body ergometer
- Versa climber
- Canoeing

As a swimmer you may be thinking that you do not want to cross train to replace your swim workouts but to cross train in conjunction with your swim workouts. Your cross-training choice will then be based on your personal circumstances, such as time of day, access to equipment, cost, and geographic variables.

9

Cross Training
for Runners

Socks, shoes, shorts, shirt, just put them on and go. Whatever your pace, whether you stride, slide, or glide with pride—walking, jogging, and running have a beautiful simplicity that active people love. Once you include cross training in your exercise program, regardless of your speed, you will soon find yourself wondering how you ever did without it. In fact, it well may be that the more dedicated you are to walking, jogging, or running, the more you will benefit from cross training. By adding new activities with different movement patterns you are bringing a healthy balance to your body. If you are susceptible to overtraining problems and injuries, you will be helping yourself considerably by replacing one or more of your regular weekly workouts with a few cross-training sessions.

Why are walking, jogging, and running such popular activities? There's a "no" explanation:

- No lessons
- No costs (except for quality footwear)
- No technology
- No time constraints
- No teammates
- No weather considerations (OK, don't go out in a hurricane)
- No special athletic prowess
- No minimum speed

Walking continues to be one of the most popular forms of exercise for thousands of Americans, and for many walkers malls have become the "field of dreams." The National Organization of Mall Walkers reports that 1,000 of the 2,300 malls nationwide offer free walking opportunities before shopping hours, usually between 6:30 A.M. and 10:00 A.M.

The Road Runners Club of America lists 460 chapters and the *National Masters News* has reported there were one hundred road races with 2,900 runners or more in 1991. With 55,793 finishers, the Lilac Bloomsday 12K in Spokane, Washington, was the largest 1991 race. The only nationally televised race, the New York City Marathon, had 25,797 runners—good for seventh place out of the top one hundred.

History of Running

Of course, at one time men and women ran for survival. To hunt, man took his makeshift spear (cross training for the upper body) and ran after some carnivore for dinner (quite sure that red meat was good for the whole family). He and his female partner would also run if some carnivore wanted to run after *them* for dinner.

As a sport, running is one of the oldest and has long been a mainstay of track-and-field competition in schools and colleges. Running for recreation, fitness, and health began on a large scale in the United States in the 1970s.

The foundation for the surge of sweat was laid in 1966 when the first of several scientific studies was presented illuminating the role exercise can play in preventing heart disease. In 1968, Dr. Ken Cooper's *Aerobics* explained exercise clearly and convincingly, serving as the launching event of the running boom. Then Frank Shorter's gold medal conquest in the 1972 Olympic marathon put a glow on distance running. Finally, in 1977, the press discovered running. Advertisers began using runners in newspaper and magazine ads. The number of runners increased from six million to twenty million in a three-year span.

The long-awaited (by exercise professionals) findings on the matter of exercise and longevity came in 1989. Dr. Steven Blair's thirteen-year study (published in the November 1989 edition of the *New England Journal of Medicine*) proved that walking briskly three times per week for thirty minutes can substantially reduce a person's chances of dying from heart disease, cancer, or other causes. This information was important to all adults, but it was particularly noteworthy for those inactive Americans who had been avoiding exercise because they thought it was for gifted athletes. Blair's conclusion that walking could make a significant difference stimulated some of the sedentary into getting away from the television.

Today, counting walkers, joggers, and runners, there are probably upward of fifty million American bipeds exercising—some fanatically, most consistently, a large number semi-regularly, and quite a few saying, "I wish I was working out more than once every two weeks!"

After thousands of years of evolution, men and women once again run to survive.

Pace

At what speed does walking become jogging; how can we differentiate between jogging and running; and while we're perambulating pace, what constitutes sprinting?

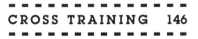

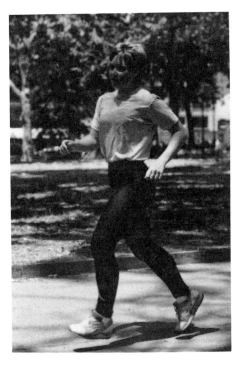

The simplicity of running explains its tremendous popularity. Many runners cross train to achieve better overall fitness.

Even the respected *Oxford English Dictionary* doesn't clarify the distinctions between jogging and running:

> *jog:* a slow measured walk, trot, or run.
> *run:* to move the legs quickly so as to go at a faster pace than walking.

When you walk, one foot is always touching the ground. Once your speed is such that your body is completely airborne during any part of the stride you are no longer walking. It is interesting to note that race-walkers frequently go faster than joggers. Even though race-walking doesn't have the vertical work component of jogging, with the swivel hip action and vigorous arm swing, race-walkers often average 5 to 6 miles per hour in competition. Jogging begins at 4.5 to 5 miles per hour for most people. The speed at which jogging is considered running is subject to argument. Some experts say that the distinction should be made at 8 to 8.5 miles per hour. Since 8.5 miles per hour represents a 7-minute mile it seems reasonable to say that this rate of advancement should be described as running.

A comment on sprinting will take us to the finish line of this talk on tempo. As luck would have it, it is easy to explain sprinting because to sprint is to run at *your* top speed, whatever that may be.

Cross Training to Improve Performance for Runners and Race-Walkers

The specificity of training principle states that to improve performance you must train as you race. To be a faster runner you must run faster in training. How then do physiologists explain the number of runners who have achieved quality performances after incorporating cross training into their workout programs? The answer to this question may be found in one or more of the following explanations:

1. Addition by subtraction.
If the runner was *overtraining*, one or two cross-training workouts per week relieves such overuse stress, leading to a better rested athlete and sounder performance.

2. Maintaining aerobic power.
If the athlete is injured to the extent that running is not possible, cardiovascular cross training prevents loss of aerobic power. When the athlete returns to running workouts, top form is regained quickly.

3. Renewed enthusiasm for training.
Serious athletes who have been training and competing for an extended period of time sometimes burn out. More than a few dedicated college swimmers have been through this experience. They recover by taking time off, swimming less when they do go back to the pool, and cross training for the pleasure of exercise *sans* goggles. Burned-out runners who have used the swimmer's formula for renewing enthusiasm have been pleased with their results.

In the May 1993 issue of *Runner's World*, Dan Bensimhon summarizes his interviews with leading exercise physiologists and elite runners. He offers cross-training programs for five different types of runners:

1. Beginning Runners (5 to 15 miles per week)
   • Mix running and cross training in equal amounts.

2. **Intermediate Runners (15 to 40 miles per week)**
   - Run two to three times as much as you cross train.

3. **Advanced Runners (more than 40 miles per week)**
   - Replace one or two of your weekly easy runs with a cross-training activity.

4. **Injury-Prone Runners (two or more running-related injuries per year)**
   - Two to four runs per week (but only one at high intensity) and the safest cross-training options you can find performed twice per week. Cross training with water activities is explained in chapter 11.

5. **General Fitness Runners (low to mid-mileage runners concerned with overall fitness)**
   - Try for two runs, two aerobic cross-training sessions that engage upper body muscles (rowing, cross-country ski machine, swimming), and two circuit training workouts, per week.

Cross Training for Variety

If you have tried all the possible routes leaving from your home, done all the local races twice, and can't find any new jogging partners, perhaps you need to cross train for the *diversion* benefits. If so, choose one of the options listed here, then get started and see how you like it.

To improve the strength and muscle tone of your upper body your top cross-training options are:

- Strength training
- Swimming
- Cross-country skiing
- AirDyne stationary bike
- Upper body ergometer
- Versa climber
- Rowing (indoors)
- Rowing (outdoors)
- Canoeing
- Rock climbing

To maintain your aerobic power while reducing repetitive motion wear and tear on your legs, your top cross-training options are:

- Water running
- Cross-country skiing
- Cycling (outdoors)
- Cycling (indoors)
- Recumbent bicycle
- Step machine
- Versa climber
- In-line skating
- Stride board workout
- Aerobic dance
- Step classes
- Social dancing

Potential Physical Fitness
Benefits Provided by Walking

Aerobic Capacity	3
Strength Upper Body	1
Strength Lower Body	2
Flexibility Upper Body	1
Flexibility Lower Body	2

These benefits assume the exerciser is following the principles of exercise as described in Chapter 3. Naturally there are some people who will gain more or less than the estimated benefit listed here.

4 = excellent	3 = good	2 = fair	1 = minimal

Potential Physical Fitness
Benefits Provided by Running

Aerobic Capacity	4
Strength Upper Body	2
Strength Lower Body	4
Flexibility Upper Body	2
Flexibility Lower Body	2

These benefits assume the exerciser is following the principles of exercise as described in Chapter 3. Naturally there are some people who will gain more or less than the estimated benefit listed here.

4 = excellent   3 = good   2 = fair   1 = minimal

As the charts above show, walking and running do not provide complete physical fitness, and it is for this reason that cross training is excellent for walkers and runners. Understand the areas you wish to work on, select the appropriate options, schedule your workouts, and start realizing the many advantages of cross training.

The Triathlon: Classic Cross Training

The triathlon is a three-part event consisting of a swim, followed immediately by a bike ride, followed immediately by a run. Triathlons are fun, they come in many different distances, and a short-course triathlon is out there for you. (The name and address of the U.S. national triathlon organization is in the appendix.)

The triathlon represents classic cross training because it uses and develops your entire body. In fact, to participate in triathlons you must use your intelligence as well. (If you enjoy your triathlon training enough to do three workouts per event per week you will be doing "triple task-specific training." You will go beyond, for example, being a swimmer who rides a bike once a week and runs now and then. You will become a *swimmer* and a *cyclist* and a *runner*.)

You may be thinking triathlons are for "aerobic animals"—those athletes with tremendous cardiorespiratory systems who can exercise for over nine hours without stopping. The short-course triathlons really are short in relation to the standard Ironman competition in which the entrants swim 2.4 miles, bike 112, and run 26.2. The short-course can include a 400-yard swim in a pool, a lake, or some other open water, a bike ride of only 10 miles, and a 3-mile run. The short-course triathlons are sometimes referred to as "sprint" triathlons. (Even the shortest triathlons are not consistent with the definition of the word *sprint* as it is applied to competitive swimming, competitive cycling, or track and field.)

The truth is, almost all triathlons are endurance events. And when you look at the exploding popularity of the sport of triathlon across the United States and throughout the world, you discover that the endurance component of the sport is a critical element. The reason is this: Each time a contestant *completes* a triathlon there is a wonderful feeling of satisfaction. Triathlons are made to order for average people who enjoy developing above-average aerobic fitness.

Begin with a sound philosophy toward your own participation. Try to put your energies toward your understanding of the events and concentrate on developing your swim/bike/run skills. Have fun planning your training program. Take pride in every workout you do. You don't even have to compete in the sport, you could do the cross-training for all the fitness benefits alone. But if you do choose to enter organized triathlons, focus on your own performance, not on the other competitors.

If you happen to be a gifted athlete and have trained diligently, you may be fortunate enough to win an award of some type. But the way to be sure you will look forward to competing is to learn to soak up the atmosphere of the event. Admire the other competitors, be impressed by the "plumbing" (gadgets to improve performance) on the newest racing bikes, watch the leaders push themselves in the run (if the course is set up that way). Enjoy the weather, the water, and the sweat. And, above all, congratulate yourself when you are done with the run whether you are an early finisher or not.

The History of Triathlon

The Mission Bay San Diego Track Club held a triathlon in 1974. But the development of triathlon to its current level of popularity is best examined by studying the evolution of the now world-famous Ironman Triathlon.

In 1977 there were three endurance events in Oahu, Hawaii—the 2.4-mile Waikiki Rough Water Swim, the Honolulu Marathon, and the Around Oahu Bicycle Race. Triathlon folklore has it that ex-Navy Captain John Collins got into an argument over who was the most fit—the long distance swimmer, the long distance runner, or the long distance cyclist. Collins suggested that the three events be run one after the other, and the Ironman Triathlon was created. Fifteen men entered the first Ironman in 1978. It was held in Oahu through 1980, at which point the event was getting too big, so race director Valerie Silk moved the race to Hawaii. Three hundred and fifty-six 1981 entrants made a large enough field for Budweiser Light to come on as a sponser beginning in 1982.

Twenty-three-year-old Julie Moss had the lead in the 1982 race with five miles to go, but she was weakening and fell to her knees. By the last fifteen yards she was literally crawling when Kathleen McCartney passed her to take the women's first place award. But, it was Moss's refusal of help and sheer guts that the ABC-TV national viewing audience admired and that gave the sport of triathlon what writer Katherine Vaz called "the stamp of validity." The drama of the McCartney/Moss finish turned the sport of triathlon into a bona fide physical endurance challenge for fitness enthusiasts all over the United States.

By 1983 approximately 250,000 participants entered over 1,000 triathlons all over the world. It is estimated that in 1991 four times as many races were offered with a half-million finishers altogether. And there are strong indications that the sport of triathlon is still growing—the U.S. National Governing Body for Triathlon reports that subscriptions to its magazine, *Triathlon Times*, increased substantially from 1987 to 1992.

In June 1991 the International Olympic Committee announced its recognition of triathlon as an Olympic sport.

The official distances will be 1.5-kilometer swim, 40-kilometer bike, and a 10-kilometer run. In miles these distances equal roughly 1, 25, and 6.2, respectively.

The International Triathlon Union is committed to promoting triathlon so that it will be granted medal sport status in prestigious international competitions.

Potential Physical Fitness Benefits Provided by Triathlon

Aerobic Capacity	4
Strength Upper Body	4
Strength Lower Body	4
Flexibility Upper Body	4
Flexibility Lower Body	3

These benefits assume the exerciser is following the principles of exercise as described in Chapter 3. Naturally there are some people who will gain more or less than the estimated benefit listed here.

4 = excellent	3 = good	2 = fair	1 = minimal

Benefits of Triathlon Training

Triathlon training clearly meets the definition of cross training presented in chapter 1: performing two or more activities within the same week. And, triathlon training can provide every benefit of cross training discussed in Chapter 2. The three different events provide stimulating variety and exciting challenge. As you do more training you will make new friends and find yourself working out at different times, in different places. Over time you will gain more and more confidence in your skill as a triathlete, and you will be pleased with your muscular development. Your aerobic capacity will begin to approach its physiological potential and you will take great pride in being able to sustain physical exertion for one or two or three hours or more, depending on your competitive goals.

But, a word of caution is necessary here. If you are not competing in triathlons to earn a living, be careful how hard and how often you train. It is possible to turn a benefit of cross training—*reduction* of injuries—into a peril associated with obsessive exercise behavior: injuries due directly to overtraining. Don't train through unusual pain. As soon as you feel you are hurt (which feels different than muscular fatigue), stop training in that event until you are completely healed. When you resume training, make adjustments in your training program to prevent getting hurt again. Remember your philosophy of triathlon training and competing: You want to be able to enjoy every workout and each competition. Listen carefully to your body and modify your training when necessary so you can have a better chance to remain injury-free year-round.

Getting Started: Swimming

You must be able to swim at least a little to participate in an actual triathlon. If you are entering the triathlon mainly to get a quality workout and to enjoy the ambience of the race, in most triathlons you can do any stroke you like. One thing you should check on is if there is a *maximum completion time* for the swim; that is, the race director may have set a time by which all swimmers must be out of the water. If the race you have selected has such a stipulation, you should time yourself to see if you are able to meet the required time. If not, more training may be in order. If you are not already doing the crawl stroke, perhaps you should switch to it. It is the fastest competitive stroke; it keeps your body in a streamlined, efficient position; it allows you to see where you are going; and the recovery phase of the stroke provides a slight rest during each arm cycle.

The crawl stroke consists of six phases, which are

explained here, but you should consider taking private lessons, a class, or joining a swim club if you truly want to improve your stroke technique.

The six phases of the crawl stroke are:

1. The Entry—your hand goes into the water.
2. The Catch—you bend your wrist slightly to catch the water
3. The Downward Press
4. The Pull—you do a sculling motion through the water bending your elbow and bringing your hand toward the midline of your body, moving your arm faster and faster.
5. The Finish—you push the water behind you as you straighten your arm.
6. The Recovery—you lift your hand and arm out of the water to set up your next stroke

The six phases follow one another to form a smooth continuous movement.

You must also pay attention to your breathing and kicking.

Breathing

Relax. The most important aspect of breathing during the crawl stroke is that you be relaxed. Inhale deeply and slowly. Exhale smoothly. The mechanics of rotating your head properly will come with practice.

Kicking

Although the crawl stroke calls for a smooth easy flutter kick that will generate only about 10 to 20 percent of your power, you do have to learn to kick properly.

The flutter kick begins at the hip joint. There should be only a slight bend in the knee as you kick, and your ankle flexibility is much more important than you might think.

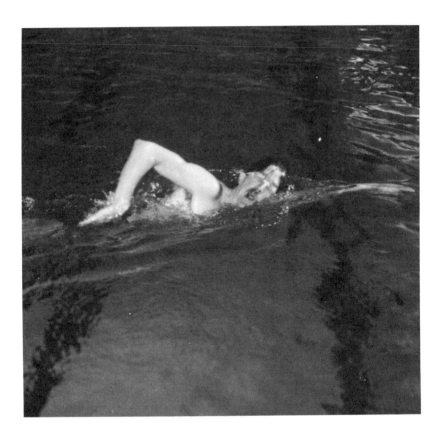

You will need access to a pool or open water to do your swim training.

Ankle Flexibility Test

To test your ankle flexibility, or plantar flexion, do this simple test. Sit down on the floor with your legs in front of you and straight. With your heel resting naturally on the floor, point your toes down toward the floor and look at the distance between your pointed toes and the floor. For most people this distance will be about five to seven inches. But if your toes could reach the floor like Olympic gold medal—winner Mark Spitz, your feet would func-

---

tion more like flippers and would provide more propulsion with less effort throughout the flutter kick.

You can improve your ankle flexibility with dry land exercises in which you point your toes forcefully, hold for ten seconds, relax for ten seconds, and repeat five times. When you get to the pool do kicking laps and swim with short rubber fins such as Zoomers or Slim Fins. Scuba fins are too heavy for the kicking you will do when lap swimming. These short fins will stretch your foot into the correct streamlined position—(don't worry, you're not cheating). You will be pushing more water and therefore forcing the kicking muscles of your legs to work harder.

Equipment

You will need a swimsuit and goggles. You can use a kickboard and fins to improve your ankle flexibility and kicking strength. Hand paddles are valuable aids for checking your stroke pattern, but don't use them more than twice a week. Pull buoys keep your body afloat so you can concentrate on your stroke.

Getting Started: Cycling

To compete, you will need a bike that fits your body and your budget. There are many triathlons that welcome non-racing bikes, so if you already have a three-speed bike or a mountain bike you can race with it. Or if you don't want to compete at all, you can do your triathlon cross-training on indoor bikes and enjoy the conditioning benefits without getting involved in the racing. If, however, you do your first race and are impressed by the dynamic-looking, serious racing bikes, you may begin thinking about purchasing one for yourself. If you decide you want to take on the challenge of triathlon training so you can complete longer bicycle segments and race faster you will

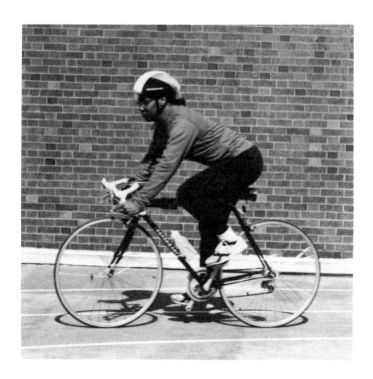

Wear layers to cycle in the cold weather.

almost certainly want to be riding on a quality racing bike.

The fit of your bike is critical to successful, efficient, pain-free riding over the long haul. The chapter 11 section "Cross Training with Wheels" explains the steps involved in proper bicycle fitting.

While You Are Riding

Keep your upper body as relaxed as possible. With time and practice you will be able to place your hands on the drops (the lower part of the handlebars) and lower your head so that your upper body is just about parallel to the ground. This is your best aerodynamic position, and the longer you can stay in it the less the wind will slow you.

Hand, Arm, and Upper Body Position

As mentioned above, keep your hands on the drops as much as possible. Don't grip the drops too hard. It's good to keep your elbows flexed. Vary your hand and arm position

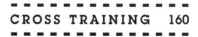

from time to time. You can shake out one arm at a time every few miles and rotate your head now and then to prevent stiffness. Again, those body parts not actively engaged in the work should be relaxed.

Pedaling Technique

One revolution occurs each time a pedal makes a complete circle, and competitive cyclists usually train and race at 90 to 110 revolutions per minute (rpms) to be physically efficient. Dave Scott, six-time winner of the Ironman Triathlon, recommends a slightly slower pedaling rate of 80 to 90 revolutions for competitive triathletes. Try training between 80 rpms and 110 rpms and see what feels best for you.

Good pedaling technique is critical to maximizing your performance and can allow you to ride more comfortably and effectively. What you need to do is to pull *back* as your pedal gets to the three o'clock position. This brings the calf and hamstring muscles into the action. The best drill for learning this is called single-leg cycling. You can set your racing bike on a wind trainer—a device used indoors that lifts the rear wheel off the ground—or you can do this drill on a stationary bike. Put one foot in the toe clips and put the other foot on a box just to the outside of the other pedal. To pedal with one foot you will find that you *must* pull the pedal back, thus you are forced to develop your pedaling technique. Set the resistance on your bike very low when you do this drill and work in intervals of thirty seconds to a minute. Do five to ten sets for each leg per workout.

Hills

To climb a gradual hill most serious cyclists slide back in the saddle and grip the handlebars close to the stem. Dave Scott, however, recommends that triathletes cycling up a hill get out of the saddle—that is, stand up on the bike. A physiologist as well as a champion triathlete, Scott believes that getting out of the saddle will allow you to use your energy more efficiently.

Sometimes, if the hill is not too steep, you may be able to stay in the same gear. Your rpms will slow down somewhat if you take the hill this way. For very steep hills you should shift to an easier gear and try to maintain your rpm pace while continuing to breathe steadily.

Brakes

To slow down safely when you are going fast it is best to use the front brake—without applying it too sharply, because you could fall over the front of your bike. The danger in hitting the back brake first is that your back wheel may slide out.

Flat Tires and Repairs

Flat tires are inevitable. Ask the bike shop personnel to teach you how to change your tires. Clincher tires have an inner tube that is easily replaced. All you have to carry in your bike bag (tied under your seat) is a set of tire irons and the correct size inner tube.

Major repairs should be done by a bicycle mechanic. As you become more and more familiar with your bike you may want to do your own minor repairs.

Bike Maintenance

Greg LeMond's *Complete Book of Bicycling* (Putnam Publishing, 1990) has a thirty-seven-page chapter detailing do-it-yourself bicycle maintenance. It is possible to get very involved in caring for your bike. If you don't naturally gravitate toward such mechanical endeavors, take your bike in for a tune-up at least once a year, for periodic adjustments, and whenever it's making a noise you don't like. Even though it is a messy job, you should at least keep your free wheel and chain clean. Keeping your tires fully inflated will reduce the possibility of a flat and give you a faster ride.

Tires

Tubular (sew-up) tires are completely enclosed and are glued to the rim of the wheel. For years tubular tires were the choice of racers because they are light and easy to change quickly. But they cost from $15 to $50 and puncture easily. Today the clincher tire is more popular than the tubular. The clincher tire sits on an inner tube similar to your car tire setup. The wider kind of clincher tire is pumped up to about 70 pounds per square inch but it's somewhat slow for serious racing. The new clinchers can be inflated to 100 to 120 pounds per square inch and are far less expensive than tubulars.

Cycling Accessories

There are many gadgets, components, and accessories to choose from to enhance your ride for speed, style, or comfort. However, if it is superior performance that you are after you should know that you cannot buy it. Your genetic potential, the quality of your training program, and your work ethic are the most important factors to analyze when you are studying how to improve your triathlon performance.

If you have an entry-level or mid-range racing bike, use it until you understand more about the sport of triathlon and racing bikes. If your bike has a decent-quality frame and fits you properly, you can think about upgrading your parts (components). Wheels are usually the component looked at first. Whether you should upgrade other components such as your derailleurs, shift levers, or pedals is a decision with which your bicycle mechanic can help.

You should have a water bottle holder and a water bottle to put in it, a pump, a seat bag (pocket pack) to hold your spare inner tube, and a cycling computer that will tell you distance traveled, miles per hour, and revolutions per minute.

Basic cycling clothes for a triathlete are a helmet (this is mandatory), stiff-soled cleated cycling shoes, padded biking shorts, padded gloves, and sunglasses.

If you find that you are turned on by the technical aspects and accessories of cycling consider getting yourself a subscription to a bicycle catalog. You will have many items from which to choose every issue.

Getting Started: Running

First of all, you don't have to run. You can do three-sport cross training by adding brisk walks to your swimming

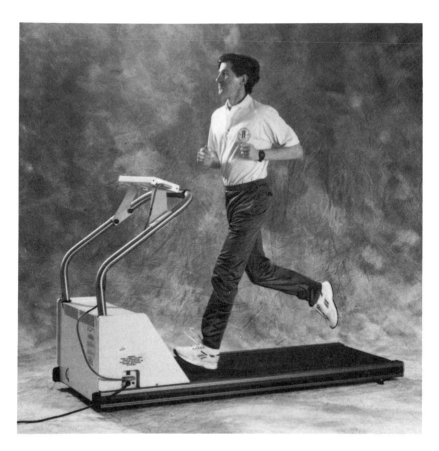

You can do many of your triathlon running workouts indoors on a treadmill.

and biking. In fact, a request to substitute walking after swimming and biking was made in the fall of 1991 by a new member of the John Jay College Triathlon Club, Eric Drucker. I explained to Eric that he was welcome to walk on the treadmill during the last segment of the Indoor Triathlon. He would be getting approximately the same physiological benefits as those entrants running the last segment, and that he should take great pride in finishing at his own pace. However, the 1991 Indoor Triathlon did not have a swim, bike, walk category. To his credit, Eric accepted the challenge of the event anyway. He jogged the last leg and had a marvelous experience.

Perhaps as the sport of triathlon expands an event will

be created for individuals who cannot or prefer not to run. Triathlon distances have been appropriately shortened for youngsters, so it seems fair that the intensity of the final segment of a triathlon could be modified as well.

Running is popular due to its simplicity. A pair of running shoes is affordable to almost everyone. Add a pair of shorts, put on a tee-shirt, and you are on your way to a running workout. After allowing for personal safety and inclement weather, you can go running almost any time of day or night. You don't have to work your schedule around the availability of a pool, and you'll never get a "flat" in your running shoe.

As you can see in the chart on page 151, running provides excellent cardiovascular fitness benefits, too. Many active people who have tried several different forms of exercise claim that running is the most effective type of workout for weight control. Of course, as the chart shows, running by itself does not provide overall physical fitness, which explains why so many runners nationwide are adding cycling, swimming, and other activities to their weekly exercise routines.

Equipment

You will need a good pair of running shoes. There is an old saying used often when referring to fixing something, "You need the right tool for the job." In the case of exercise you need the right equipment for your sport, and in the case of running you should have footwear designed specifically for running. Today's running shoes are designed to protect your foot, your ankle, and your knee from injury. If you try to run regularly in footwear meant for some other sport you are unnecessarily increasing your risk of injury. Further, a quality running shoe will feel better than any other, and finally, if speed becomes important to you, you will want less weight on your feet as you run. Quality running shoes are both durable and lightweight.

When selecting running shoes the single most important factor to be aware of is comfort. Your running shoes should feel good as soon as you lace them up and move around. The different brand-name companies make running shoes with slightly different contours, so try on a few different pairs to see which are most comfortable on your feet. Then talk to the salesman about your probable weekly mileage, the relative weight of the different brands (to achieve your best performance you will want to purchase the lightest shoe you can afford), and price range.

Your Running Workouts

Little by little—that is how you will build up to your running goal, whether that goal is one mile or 26.2 miles. Imagine you are going out for your first run. Let's see if you are ready.

First Run Checklist
- - - - - - - - - - - - -

1. Do you have a quality pair of running shoes?
2. Do you have a pair of white cotton sweat socks? (They will provide cushioning and absorb sweat without changing the color of your feet.)
3. Do you have an appropriate pair of exercise shorts?
4. Are you wearing an athletic supporter or a jogging bra?
5. And do you have your tee-shirt or singlet (an exercise shirt designed for runners without sleeves)?

Weather Conditions

Your attire will be affected by the weather when you run outside. If it's cold, wear layers such as a tee-shirt, sweat shirt, warm-up jacket. Or, if you can afford the synthetic fiber shirts and running tights made of Lycra, which are form-fitting, you may enjoy a wicker effect—your perspiration evaporates through the material while much of your body heat is retained. Another option if it is cold is to wear thermal underwear and a second pair of socks. Wear a woolen hat to protect your ears and keep your head warm; wear gloves to protect your hands. (I used to wear a pair of socks on my hands, but my wife said I looked too strange. Litna bought me an inexpensive pair of gloves to wear instead, but I still wear the socks on my hands sometimes, anyway.)

Cold weather should not stop you from running outside if you dress properly. Start slowly and finish slowly and you will soon find your outdoor runs invigorating.

Running in the Heat

If it's hot outside you should take some steps to protect yourself from the heat. Use a lotion with a high SPF (Sun Protection Factor) to prevent sunburn. Wear a runner's cap with a visor to keep some of the sun off your face. Wear a lightweight, light-colored tee-shirt or singlet, shorts, and anklet socks (or cuff regular socks) so the perspiration on your legs can evaporate freely. Perspiration is your body's method for cooling itself. Wearing rubberized suits is not a good idea. These suits do not let your perspiration evaporate, making it difficult for your skin to breathe. This can lead to overheating and may even be dangerous.

While exercising in the heat you should take care to maintain your body fluid level. Hydrate your body by drinking water before you go out to run in the heat. Do not wait until you feel thirsty to have a drink, because by that time you have already begun to dehydrate. Our thirst mechanism notifies us too late for it to be used as the drink indicator. If you are doing a workout on your own try to arrange a route that allows you to drink more water as you run. During a race on a hot day there should be a water station every few miles. Be sure to drink a few ounces at every opportunity. On a hot day you may have to adjust your distance goal and your pace. After your workout drink more water and replenish your body's minerals by having bananas, watermelon, cantaloupe, carrots, or tomatoes. You may want to try a runner's drink that has replacement electrolytes and minerals.

Finding Time to Train: Workout Options

It can be challenging to find the time for your new cross training workouts. There are ideas which you may find helpful in Chapter 7, page 89, Cross Training to Open New Time of Day Workout Options.

If you want to get some of the cross-training benefits of swim-bike-run workouts without entering a triathlon event, you can do so by adding one workout of each of the two new activities to your primary workout. If you swim three times a week now, just schedule one bike workout per week (20 to 60 minutes, indoors or outdoors) and one run per week (20 to 30 minutes, indoors or outdoors), and you will be cross training beautifully.

On the other hand, if you are excited about trying a real triathlon, your next step is to write out a training schedule. The planning for Your First Triathlon chart on page 169 will help you with this. Make copies of the chart if you think it will be useful to you. Then look at the Fifty-Day Training Program on page 170 and get a sense of the time involved per workout and the number of workouts per week.

Your First Triathlon:
From Locating It to Loving It

Reasonable first triathlon race goals: finish, don't get hurt, enjoy yourself. Your approach to race events is far more important than your time. Just as it is not necessary to sound like Billy Joel to enjoy playing the piano, it is not necessary to race like Mark Allen (1992 Ironman winner) to enjoy participating in a full-fledged triathlon. If you practice a piece on the piano until you play it well you are proud. By the same measure, if you do the training necessary to complete a triathlon, whatever the distance, you should take pride in finishing. This brings us to the essence of a successful race event: preparation. If you prepare properly by training intelligently you will be successful and enjoy your race.

Now that you have a sound philosophy for entering competitive traithlons, you should find a short-course event appropriate to your ability. (See the appendix for triathlon organization information.) Once you have your race picked out you will know the distances involved for each leg. Then you can modify the training times suggested in the Fifty-Day Training Program to meet your needs. If your training sessions go well you should be able to say to yourself, "I know I can handle this triathlon because I have done the equivalent distances during my workouts."

Planning for Your First Triathlon
A Fifty Day Training Program

WEEK	One	Two	Three	Four	Five	Six	Seven
DAY							
Monday	Swim 10:00	Swim 15:00	Swim 20:00	Swim 20:00	Swim 25:00	Swim 30:00	Swim 15:00
Tuesday	Bike 30:00	Bike 30:00	Bike 20:00	Bike 45:00	Bike 30:00	Bike 30:00	Run 20:00
Wednesday	OFF	OFF	OFF	OFF	OFF	OFF	OFF
Thursday	Run 15:00	Run 15:00	Swim 15:00	Swim 15:00	Swim 20:00	Run 40:00	Bike 15:00
Friday	Swim 15:00	Swim 15:00	Run 25:00	Run 30:00	Run 35:00	Swim 20:00	Swim 15:00
Saturday	Bike 30:00	Bike 35:00	Bike 40:00	Bike 45:00	Bike 50:00	Bike 60:00	OFF*
Sunday	OFF	OFF	OFF	OFF	Run 15:00	Run 20:00	RACE DAY!
Workouts per week =	5	5	5	5	6	6	4
Training Time	Swim = 25 Bike = 60 Run = 15	Swim = 30 Bike = 65 Run = 15	Swim = 35 Bike = 40 Run = 45	Swim = 35 Bike = 90 Run = 30	Swim = 45 Bike = 50 Run = 80	Swim = 50 Bike = 90 Run = 60	Swim = 30 Bike = 30 Run = 20

Adapt training time and distance to the distances of your first triathlon. For example, If your event involves a quarter mile swim, and you find you can do that in 11:00 minutes (or less), you don't have to do training swims of 25:00 and 30:00 minutes.

*Dave Scott recommends a light workout the day before the race. Try both methods of preparation and see which you prefer.

Planning for Your First Triathlon
A Fifty Day Training Program

WEEK	One	Two	Three	Four	Five	Six	Seven
DAY							
Monday							
Tuesday							
Wednesday							
Thursday							
Friday							
Saturday							
Sunday							

Workouts per week =

Training Time	Swim =	Swim =	Swim =	Swim =	Swim =	Swim =
	Bike =	Bike =	Bike =	Bike =	Bike =	Bike =
	Run =	Run =	Run =	Run =	Run =	Run =

Final Week Preparations

- Were you expecting an acceptance letter? If it has not arrived contact race officials.
- Do you have travel directions to the race?
- What is the weather forecast? Bring race clothing appropriate to the temperature expected.
- Does your bicycle need fine-tuning?
- You should be tapering your training; that is, cutting back on time, distance, and intensity to allow your muscles to regain full strength.
- Do not do the whole course the day before the race. You may want to look the course over or drive through parts of it so you will have a sense of where the hills and turns are.

The Night before the Triathlon

Lay out everything you need to take and make a checklist for yourself.

_____ Directions

_____ Race numbers (to wear on your bike and during the run)

Swim Gear

_____ Swimsuit

_____ Wet suit (wear if water is 75 degrees or lower. Another benefit of the wet suit is faster swim time—it makes you more buoyant in the water.)

_____ Goggles (bring an extra pair)

_____ Swim cap

Swim-to-Bike-Transition Gear

_____ Extra water bottle (in addition to the water bottle on your bike)

_____ Hand towel for wiping feet

_____ Bike shoes (although for short races some triathletes wear running shoes during the bike phase and save changing time)

_____ Powder for inside of shoes

Bike Gear

_____ Water bucket (to rinse off sand)

_____ Sunglasses

_____ Shirt

_____ Helmet

_____ Bike gloves

Bike-to-Run-Transition

_____ Running shoes

_____ Water

_____ Hat or visor

Triathlon Morning

A typical starting time for a triathlon is 7:00 A.M. or 8:00 A.M. You should be out of bed at least two hours prior to the race start to allow your body and mind time to get ready.

For a short-course triathlon you could have a regular balanced dinner around eight the night before and not eat anything in the morning. If you do want to eat in the morning, try a banana or two *at least* two hours prior to the race start. Do not eat anything within one hour of the race start.

It's a good idea to do a pre-race warm-up. It will shunt blood to the muscles that will be working, prepare your respiratory and circulatory systems, and increase your flexibility and overall alertness.

Your pre-race warm-up should be done about thirty minutes before the race begins and at a very low intensity. If the water is not too cold (75 degrees is cold) swim a little and get a feel for the water. Swimming 100 to 200 yards should be fine if your swim leg is under one mile. Do not let yourself get tired.

Cycle about ten minutes in a low gear at about 10 miles per hour. Leave your bike in a low gear when you put it on the rack.

Jog 400 to 800 yards, very slowly.

Do a few minutes of stretching using your normal stretching routine and once you are warm, stay warm.

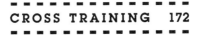

Triathlon!

The Swim

During the swim, breathe easy, breathe with each arm cycle, and stay relaxed. You may find it helpful to change strokes now and then for ten seconds. If you can do the breast stroke you will be able to see where you are going; a little backstroke will loosen your shoulder muscles. While it is legal to swim directly behind someone else in the swim ("drafting" is the term used to describe this action) you may not necessarily want to draft in the water. If you are drafting during the swim someone else is navigating—what if he or she goes off course? Also, you are letting this person establish pace for you, and it may not be the best pace for your swim ability.

Swim-to-Bike-Transition

Jog easily as you leave the water. Let the blood circulate to your leg muscles. Take a drink of water if it's available, or take a few sips of your own extra water bottle. Depending on the weather conditions you may need to do nothing more than put on your bike shoes (or running shoes) and your helmet and go! If the sun is strong you may need to put on a shirt and sunglasses.

The Bike

Maneuver your bike through the transition area carefully. Once you are on your bike Begin in a low or medium gear at 70 to 80 revolutions per minute for the first 100 to 200 yards. It will take a while for your blood supply to move to your muscles. In a few minutes you will settle into a steady leg rhythm. Get comfortable on the bike and breathe easily. Set a speed that you feel you can sustain through the end of the bike without getting out of breath. As you head into the last half-mile you can prepare your legs and feet for the run by shifting into a lower gear, standing on the pedals and stretching, moving your toes inside your shoes, and varying your pedaling routine slightly (try moving your knees in and out and take turns pushing hard with each leg).

When you are about 75 to 100 yards from the transition area loosen the toe clips and shoe straps or laces to allow blood to flow more readily to your feet. Undo the chin strap on your helmet. Think about where you will be putting your bike after you are in the transition area.

Bike-to-Run-Transition

Put your bike on the rack. Slowly sit down and put on your running shoes. Drink some water. Shuffle, don't sprint, out of the transition area.

The Run

Use a short stride for a little while. When you feel you are ready to go faster, take faster steps but do not lengthen your stride until you feel you have good flexibility in your quadriceps, hamstrings, and hips. Swing your arms gently, shake out your hands a few times, and if you feel up to it, take in the scenery.

You Did It!

Congratulate yourself—you finished! Keep moving by walking for a few minutes. Drink some fluid and have something to eat. Get out of the sun; take a massage if it's available. Put on a dry tee-shirt or light jacket and stretch—very gently.

When you get home you may find it satisfying to write down your impressions of your first competitive triathlon. Did you find it to be as you expected? What was easy? What was hard? Did you pace yourself well? Do you feel you want to do another triathlon one day? Will you train the same way you did for your first triathlon? If you enjoyed the physical and mental preparations for your first triathlon, you are now looking forward to many years of rewarding cross training.

The Indoor Triathlon

Could a triathlon be held indoors within a predetermined time frame? Several members of John Jay College's Physical Education Department set out to answer this question in spring 1989.

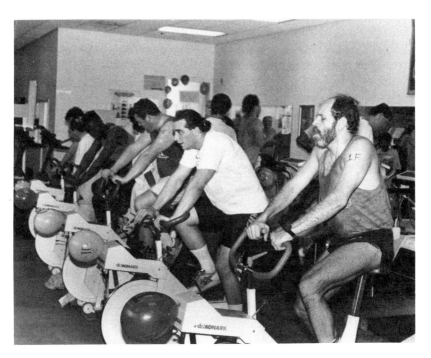

These cyclists are working hard during the middle segment of their indoor triathlon.
(Photo credit to Mikki McNulty.)

At John Jay, the Cardiovascular Fitness Center has six Monark cycle ergometers and six Quinton treadmills, along with a full complement of other exercise equipment. Factor in the 25-yard, five-lane NCAA regulation pool and the three components needed to hold a triathlon were on hand. But how could we organize the indoor event so that it would be completed within the one and a half hours scheduled for intramural activities?

The triathlon we created required the entrants to do each segment for 10 minutes, and we put five competitors in each heat (one per swim lane). At the end of each 10-minute swim, competitors had 5 minutes "transition" time to get their sneakers and tee-shirts on and get themselves into the elevator for the ride from the basement-level pool to the sixth floor. After the 10-minute bike at workload 1.5 kiloponds (1.5 kp is a fairly light workload), the competitors had one minute for the second transition. In other words, they had one minute to get on the treadmill for a 10-minute walk, jog, or run.

Total distance traveled in the allotted time are calculated for each competitor. To give the swim equal weight with the run, the number of yards completed in the pool is multiplied by four and then converted to mileage. The Monark cycle ergometer has a trip odometer that can be reset to zero after each rider and gives total kilometers for each ride. The total kilometers for the 10-minute stationary bike ride are converted into mileage, too, and the treadmill console provides a mileage readout to the hundredth of a mile. The distances traveled for each segment are added up and the contestant who traveled the farthest is the overall winner.

If you have access to an exercise facility with a pool, bikes, and a treadmill or track, you can set up your own indoor triathlon. It is a well-balanced aerobic workout, and you might just find it as exhilarating as the John Jay College finishers.

11

Cross Training
With Activities:
Twenty Choices

Several of the choices presented in this chapter are competitive sports. However, swimming, cycling, in-line skating, canoeing, rowing, and orienteering can be performed noncompetitively for the pleasure of the activity and the accompanying physical fitness benefits.

Each of the twenty activities is described so that you will learn what cross-training benefits the activity offers and how to begin incorporating it into your weekly exercise routine.

Cross Training in Water:
Never Let Them See You Sweat

Water is a magnificent medium. When you are in up to your chin, water's buoyancy allows you to weigh only about 10 percent of your weight on land. Thus, while moving your limbs in the water you are working several muscles groups but not subjecting your joints to the stress experienced during a land workout.

Cross Training with Swimming

Men and women have been swimming for thousands of years. There are records of swimming competitions taking place in Japan in 36 B.C. Olympic swimming events began in 1896 and the International Swimming Federation was founded in 1908.

The stroke recognized earliest was the breaststroke, next came the sidestroke, and at the end of the nineteenth century the crawl stroke was developed. The turned-head breathing pattern of the crawl was refined by Jam Handy in 1905, just prior to the advent of the backstroke, and in the 1930s the butterfly came on the scene. If you are able to master more than one stroke you can cross train within the sport of swimming because each stroke works the muscles and rotates the joints differently.

As the chart on page 139 shows, swimming is an excellent cross-training choice for physical development because it provides balanced overall fitness.

Getting Started: Swimming

If you are a nonswimmer you probably know you are going to need a few lessons. You may be glad to know there are many adults just like you who managed to get through childhood without learning to swim, then go on to take classes and end up swimming beautifully. Curtis Alitz was an All-American runner at West Point. In 1984 he decided he wanted to try triathlons and took swim lessons in his late twenties. Now he swims a mile easily.

One of the best things you can do to help yourself become a better swimmer is to learn how to do a self-evaluation of your stroke. Knowing exactly what you are supposed to be doing as your hand moves through the water and as you turn your head for a breath will allow you to continue to improve your stroke long after you have finished your formal class. Performing any stroke properly requires much practice and concentration. In fact, most swim instructors break a stroke down into components and recommend you practice them separately at the beginning of each workout.

For example, if you are learning the front crawl (freestyle), you might do a swim workout like this:

	Minutes
1. Dry land stretching (see chapter 4)	3:00
2. Bobbing—take a breath, then put your head underwater and exhale. Repeat 10 times.	1:00
3. Flutter kick 50 to 100 yards with paddle board. It's all right to rest after each lap if necessary.	2:00–4:00
4. Breathing concentration drill—use pull buoys (styrofoam floats) for your legs so you don't have to think about kicking and swim 50 to 100 yards, concentrating on breathing properly.	1:30–3:00
5. Stroke concentration drill—again use the pull buoys for your legs and swim 50 to 100 yards concentrating on your stroke technique.	1:30–3:00
6. Rest. Repeat upper body stretches.	1:00–2:00
7. Continuous swim. Put the three components together and swim as many laps as you can. Stop when you are tired, rest as necessary. Your goal is to swim 5 minutes continuously, then 10, and finally 20.	5:00–20:00
8. Cooldown—swim a lap or two very slowly if you can. Then repeat your upper body stretches while taking a few deep breaths to help lower your heart rate.	3:00

Total Time: 18:00–35:00

Exercise Prescription for a Beginning Swimmer

• *Intensity*: Due to the cooling effect of water, your heart rate during your swim workout will tend to be 10 to 15 percent lower than it would be for the same amount of work on land. But you should be aware that as a beginning swimmer, you will usually be working very hard because your stroke is not yet efficient. In short, concentrate on your form and not on your target heart rate until you have the ability to swim at different speeds with relative ease.

• *Frequency*: Since you are swimming as a cross-training alternative, once or twice a week is fine. If you decide to become more skilled or learn other strokes, you may want to swim more often.

• *Duration*: The less efficient you are in the water, the harder you work per lap, and the sooner you will be tired. So, try for ten or fifteen minutes of actual swimming, whether it be drills or complete strokes, and work your way up to a twenty-minute continuous swim.

• *Progression*: Once you have mastered the mechanics enough to take in oxygen by breathing properly while swimming, it's only a matter of practice before you will be swimming laps continuously. Try to work your way up to a twenty-minute swim.

Cross Training with Water Exercises

Exercising in the water has been labeled many times, including: aquacize, aquamotion, aquaerobics, aquadance, hydroaerobics, hydroslimnastics, and water exercise techniques. (An excellent introduction to water exercise can be found in Jane Katz's *Swim 30 Laps in 30 Days*, Perigee Books, 1991). The chart below shows the potential physical fitness benefits of water exercise.

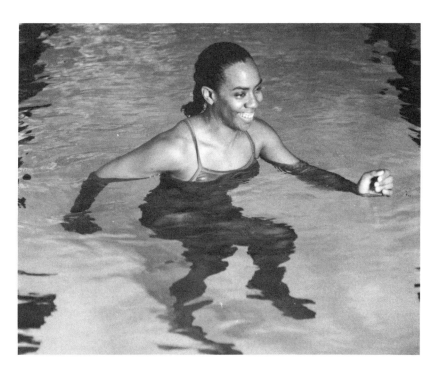

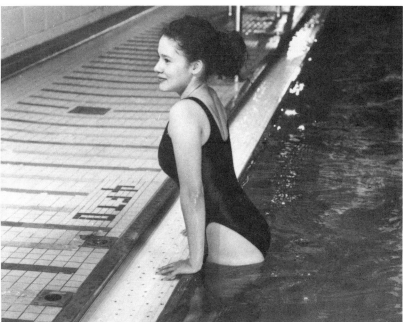

Running in place and pool pushups are but two of many invigorating water exercises.

Potential Physical Fitness
Benefits Provided by Water Exercise

Aerobic Capacity	3
Strength Upper Body	3
Strength Lower body	2
Flexibility Upper Body	2
Flexibility Lower Body	3

These benefits assume the exerciser is following the principles of exercise as described in Chapter 3. Naturally there are some people who will gain more or less than the estimated benefit listed here.

4 = excellent   3 = good   2 = fair   1 = minimal

Movement in water has virtually no impact. The chances of bone or joint injuries are minimal. Water offers four times the resistance of air, so you can work on muscle groups such as the inner and outer thigh muscles that are not easy to strengthen on land.

Exercising in the water can provide cardiovascular fitness, upper and lower body muscles tone and flexibility, and muscular endurance. For many people water exercising is more comfortable than land exercise because the water cools the body—you sweat but you don't realize it.

Water exercise is particularly good for you if you are overweight, if you have joint or limb problems, or arthritis. One famous basketball player who used water exercise to rescue his career from a serious knee injury is former New York Knickerbocker Bernard King. Future NBA Hall of Famer Larry Bird used water running for conditioning purposes and as therapy for his back. And when long jump record holder Mike Powell injured himself in the summer of 1992 he, too, turned to water exercise to stay in shape until his hamstring healed.

Getting Started: Water Exercise

Besides your swimsuit, all you need is a class with a good instructor. Try contacting your local college, Y, or health club. Evaluate the class by asking: Did the instructor take you through a gradual warm-up, a main bout of exercise, where you could feel your heart working, and a cooldown? Were most of your major muscle groups utilized? Did you spend some time stretching? And finally, did you enjoy the class? If you can answer yes to all of these questions you are set to do your water exercise. (If you can't find a class, you can do a solo workout as described in Jane Katz's *30 Laps in 30 Days.*)

Exercise Prescription: Water Exercises

• *Intensity*: Remember that the water's cooling effect will keep your heart rate 10 to 15 percent lower than the equivalent amount of land exercise, so you may not reach your target heart rate zone, even though you feel you are working hard. You might want to use the Rating of Perceived Exertion Scale (page 16) to evaluate your intensity. Your RPE score during water exercise should be about the same as your RPE score during your land workouts. If it is much higher, consider adjusting your pace within the water exercise class.

• *Frequency*: As a cross-training option, you would be likely to do water exercise workouts once or twice a week.

• *Duration*: Water exercise classes typically last 45 minutes to an hour.

• *Progression*: At some pools you can "graduate" to an advanced water exercise class. Or you may just work harder within each class as you feel yourself getting stronger.

Cross Training with Water Running

Thirty years ago, Indiana University track coach Sam Bell had his injured runners running in the water. By wearing water-ski vests they were able to stay afloat in deep water and work their leg muscles through the full running range of motion without the stress generated by land workouts.

Elite runners such as Joan Benoit-Samuelson, winner of

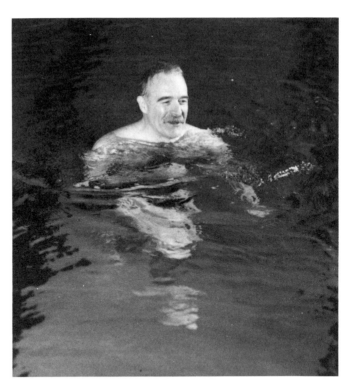

Deep water running's popularity is increasing rapidly because it allows you to maintain an excellent level of aerobic conditioning while placing a minimum of stress on your joints.

the 1984 Women's Olympic Marathon, have been running in deep water for years. Today, recreational athletes from many different sports are discovering water running as a method of cross training.

Deep water running is easier to do than swimming because you don't have to master stroke technique or rhythmic breathing. You simply do as the name suggests— you run in the deep water with a flotation device that helps keep your head above water. However, water running is not for runners only by any means. Whatever your primary activity, if you have a lower body injury caused by a muscle imbalance or overtraining, you can probably benefit from water running.

Potential Physical Fitness
Benefits Provided by Deep Water Running

Aerobic Capacity	4
Strength Upper Body	2
Strength Lower Body	3
Flexibility Upper Body	2
Flexibility Lower Body	3

These benefits assume the exerciser is following the principles of exercise as described in Chapter 3. Naturally there are some people who will gain more or less than the estimated benefit listed here.

4 = excellent   3 = good   2 = fair   1 = minimal

Getting Started: Deep Water Running

Deep water running classes are being offered in some cities across the United States and a class is a good way to begin. If there are no deep water running classes offered in your neighborhood, you can still get started easily. You will need your swimsuit, a water floatation device (the Aqua-jogger is designed for deep water running), and a body of water deep enough to permit to do a running motion without your feet hitting the bottom of the pool.

Exercise Prescription: Deep Water Running

Just as for any other workout, start slowly. Do an easy jogging motion for the first five minutes to warm your muscles.

• *Intensity*: Check your pulse and remember that for the same effort as you would expend on land your heart rate will be approximately 15 percent lower in water. If you try for heart rates in the 130–140 zone when you run on land (or treadmill) then you want to bring your heart rate up to 110–119 while doing water running.

• *Duration*: A class may last 45 minutes, but during your first few weeks 20 minutes of actual water running will enough for a quality workout.

• *Frequency*: If you are cross training with water running in order to maintain conditioning for a running activity you must do at least three workouts per week. For high levels of cardiovascular performance four or more workouts per week may be necessary.

• *Progression*: Establish your goals and the appropriate progression will follow. Are you doing water running to develop or maintain long distance running ability? If so, you will have to increase your time running in the water. If your sport demands frequent stops interspersed with high-intensity aerobic exercise—a racquet sport for example—then you must work up to a workout that mimics that type of action. Interval training would be an excellent choice.

There is more technique involved than you might think if you want to get a good workout from your water running class. Listen to your instructor. Once you feel you have mastered the techniques involved you can consider fitting in a few water running workouts without the group.

Aerobic Cross Training with Indoor Equipment: "You Gotta Try New Things"

Come in from the cold—or the heat or the rain—and try aerobic cross training with indoor equipment. The machines are easy to learn, lots of fun, and each of the eight apparatuses described here provides cardiovascular fitness while exercising the muscles at different angles. This is important because varying the rotation of the joints and the movement pathways of the muscles greatly reduces the possibility of overuse injuries.

Versions of these machines are being installed in homes all across the country because people know they will do their workouts more consistently when it is easy and convenient. If you are going to cross train on any of this equipment in a commercial fitness center or health club there are some questions you should raise before you take out a membership. What qualifications and credentials does the staff have? Is there a medical screening, fitness testing, exercise prescription entrance process? Are instructors available to teach you proper use of the equipment? Are you impressed with the appearance and cleanliness of the facility? If you are satisfied with the answers to these questions you are more likely to be satisfied with your workouts.

Cross-Country Ski Machines

The cross-country ski machine is often touted as a wonderful overall physical fitness workout because the cardiovascular system is trained at the same time as the *legs and arms* are toned. This claim is valid assuming you are working out on one of the better cross-country ski machines. But even the best models do not simulate all of the movements involved in outdoor cross-country skiing. What you will do is replicate the pull-and-glide motion used on level terrain when cross-country skiing outdoors. Second, because the pull (arms) and glide (legs) motion is somewhat different than movements we perform in everyday living or popular sport, it may take a couple of tries to feel comfortable with the machine.

Learning tip: Practice the leg motion without the arms first. After you are comfortable with the legs, then take the handles and add the arm motion. When you are doing the combined motion remember it is like walking, in that the right arm and the left leg should be going in the same direction at the same time.

Exercise Prescription: Cross-Country Ski Machines

• *Intensity*: You should keep in mind that during your first few cross-country ski machine workouts you will probably be concentrating on learning the motions. You may find yourself stopping and starting over or going fairly slow. It is OK if your heart rate does not go up into your target heart rate zone during this learning phase. Do a few five-minute practice sessions. Once you have mastered the motion, you will be able to ski faster and harder and take your heart rate up into your target heart rate zone.
• *Frequency*: If you wish to ski smoothly sooner, ski

several times per week. Otherwise, just add one or two ski machine workouts to your weekly schedule.

• "*Duration:* Your goal should be to work your way up to 20 minutes continuously.

Potential Physical Fitness
Benefits Provided by Cross-Country Ski Machine

Aerobic Capacity	4
Strength Upper Body	3
Strength Lower Body	3
Flexibility Upper Body	3
Flexibility Lower Body	3

These benefits assume the exerciser is following the principles of exercise as described in Chapter 3. Naturally there are some people who will gain more or less than the estimated benefit listed here.

4 = excellent   3 = good   2 = fair   1 = minimal

Cross Training with Indoor Exercise Bikes

Indoor exercise bikes can be grouped into four categories: cycle ergometers, computerized bikes, bikes that offer upper body action, and recumbent bikes.

Cycling performed on any of the indoor exercise bikes can provide aerobic fitness benefits. The lower body muscle group that is worked heavily involves the quadriceps. If you have toe-clip pedals and you concentrate on the upstroke (pulling the pedal up) you can work the hamstring muscle group. Competitive cyclists force themselves to work on this aspect of cycling technique by pedaling with one foot at a time.

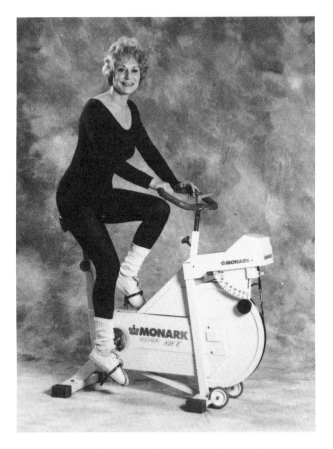

Having a stationary bike in your home increases your time of day workout options.

Ergometer comes from the Greek *ergon* (work) and *metron* (measurement). Cycle ergometers have one wheel, usually called the flywheel. Each time the exerciser pushes a pedal one full revolution the rider has moved a point on the flywheel rim an exact distance. Thus, one of the two advantages of cycle ergometers is the ability to measure your workload precisely. This allows you to set a specific exercise prescription and compare heart rate response from one workout to another. Secondly, whether on a cycle ergometer or a regular bicycle, cycling is a nonweight-bearing activity that is easier on your joints than any running activity.

Potential Physical Fitness
Benefits Provided by Cycling (Stationary Bike)

Aerobic Capacity	4
Strength Upper Body	1
Strength Lower Body	4
Flexibility Upper Body	2
Flexibility Lower Body	2

These benefits assume the exerciser is following the principles of exercise as described in Chapter 3. Naturally there are some people who will gain more or less than the estimated benefit listed here.

4 = excellent   3 = good   2 = fair   1 = minimal

Computerized bikes usually have colorful consoles that are stimulating to look at and provide feedback throughout your workout, such as minutes elapsed, intensity level, revolutions per minute, caloric expenditure, and exercise heart rate.

There is at least one bike on the market with handles you can push and pull while you pedal, offering upper body exercise. The Air Dyne indoor bike mainly works the anterior deltoid and the triceps muscles when you push the handles.

The recumbent bike seat distributes your weight differently than the traditional bike seat by firmly supporting your back. Recumbents are more comfortable than regular bikes for most exercisers.

Exercise Prescription: Indoor Exercise Bikes

• *Intensity*: It is easy to check your pulse while you are riding. If your concentration has faded and you are falling below your target heart rate zone you have two options: (1) You can renew your efforts to work in your target heart rate zone by pedaling faster, or (2) you can continue pedaling at the heart rate that is below target rate to develop endurance and burn extra calories.

• *Frequency*: As a cross-training alternative you need only ride once or twice per week. If you find you enjoy indoor cycling and have the time to do more than two workouts weekly, go for it.

• *Duration*: Work your way up to 20 minutes continuously.

• *Progression*: If you are finding your heart rate below target zone, you can then increase either your revolutions per minute (ride faster) or the resistance on the pedals (this will strengthen your quadriceps more than riding faster).

Cross Training with Slide Boards

You begin standing in the middle of a rectangular board approximately 4' x 8'. With knees bent you push off one leg and glide on the opposite foot toward the outer edge of the mat, change directions smoothly and repeat.

Slide boarding provides a complete cardiovascular workout. The motion utilizes leg muscles needed for cross-country skiing, downhill skiing, ice-skating, in-line skating, basketball, racquet sports, and soccer.

Slide boards are a recent addition to exercise facilities and home training programs. Some models have already been refined. Before making a purchase, find a board so you can do a three-minute trail workout. See if your stride fits and whether you will enjoy slide boarding.

Body Slide ($49.95) has received good ratings from fitness experts and is ordered by calling 800-652-5544. Also available are the NordicSport Lateral Trainer by Kneedspeed ($129.95), 800-892-2174; and the Training Camp Slide ($169–$199), 800-238-5241.

And finally, you should know about the Nordic Track Aerobic Cross-Trainer ($1,199.95), which provides you with a treadmill, a cross-country ski machine, and a stair climber. In its current form the Aerobic Cross-Trainer offers an intense workout. It may be wise to try a workout before purchasing the machine. The Aerobic Cross-Trainer can be ordered from Nordic Track at 800-421-5910.

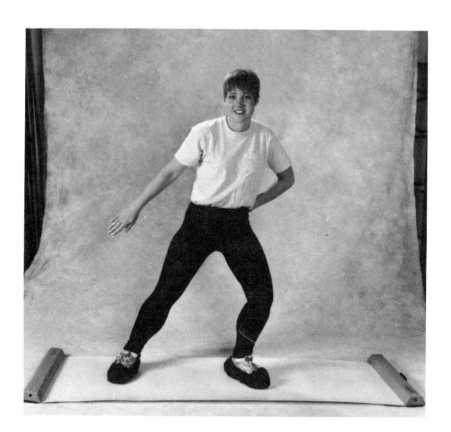

Slide boarding, also known as lateral training, is a good indoor aerobic cross training option.

Exercise Prescription: Slide Boards

• *Intensity*: Five minutes after you are sliding smoothly check your pulse. If your heart rate is below your target zone try sliding a little faster. If your heart rate is above your target zone decide whether you will be able to continue at your current intensity for fifteen more minutes. If not, slow down.

• *Frequency*: As a weekly option one or two slide boarding workouts per week will be fine. If you wish to do seasonal cross training with your slide board and maintain cardioascular fitness you will need to do three or more workouts per week.

• *Duration*: Work up to twenty minutes continuously.

• *Progression*: You can set goals for slides per minute (pace) or time.

Potential Physical Fitness
Benefits Provided by Slide Boarding

Aerobic Capacity	4
Strength Upper Body	2
Strength Lower Body	3
Flexibility Upper Body	2
Flexibility Lower Body	3

These benefits assume the exerciser is following the principles of exercise as described in Chapter 3. Naturally there are some people who will gain more or less than the estimated benefit listed here.

4 = excellent   3 = good   2 = fair   1 = minimal

Cross Training with Jumping Rope

Jumping rope is an excellent cross-training alternative because it provides aerobic conditioning, lower body muscle tone, and overall muscular endurance. Boxers have cross trained by jumping rope for many years because it simulates the physical demands of boxing. When you jump rope you are on the balls of your feet and your hands are moving all the time. . . . *Note:* If you have not been doing any exercise lately or are overweight be sure to check with your physician before jumping rope, because even jumping at a slow pace can be a vigorous workout.

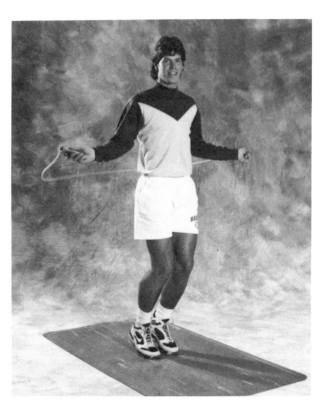

Jumping rope provides the sense of mastering a skill, is inexpensive, and rates high for overall physical fitness because both your upper and lower body are working.

These days, most jump ropes are made of rope, plastic, or leather and have ball bearings in the handles for smooth rope rotation. A jump rope may well be the least expensive piece of cardiovascular training equipment you can purchase—even a top of the line model from your local sporting goods store should cost less than $15 and will last for years.

To check your rope for the proper length, stand on the rope with your legs together and bring the handles up alongside your body. They should reach to within 6 inches or so of the top of your shoulders.

Is jumping rope easy to learn? Here is a step-by-step method for learning how to jump rope:

Potential Physical Fitness
Benefits Provided by Jumping Rope

Aerobic Capacity	4
Strength Upper Body	3
Strength Lower Body	4
Flexibility Upper Body	3
Flexibility Lower Body	2

These benefits assume the exerciser is following the principles of exercise as described in Chapter 3. Naturally there are some people who will gain more or less than the estimated benefit listed here.

4 = excellent   3 = good   2 = fair   1 = minimal

Phase I: Jumping without the Rope

1. Put the rope down. Pretend you are holding the rope handles and move your wrists in small forward circles while your hands are near your sides.
2. Begin jumping and try to go only about two inches off the ground per jump. This drill will help you avoid a common error of beginning jumpers—jumping too high per jump and getting very tired quickly.
3. Jump for 30 seconds at a time and do 5 to 10 sets. Rest as needed between sets.
4. Repeat this workout two times before moving to Phase II.

Phase II: Timing Drill

1. Take both handles in one hand and hold the rope about a third of the way down in the other hand. Begin jumping as you did in Phase I, about two inches off the ground per jump.

2. Now, controlling the rope with the hand that is not holding the handles, swing the rope along your side so that as your feet leave the ground the rope touches the ground. This drill gives you a sense of the timing of your jump.
3. Do two sessions of the timing drill.

Phase III: adding the Rope

1. Hold one handle in each hand and step over the rope so that the swag of the rope is laying on the ground just behind your heels.
2. Lift the handles simultaneously in a smooth, quick motion thus flipping the rope over your head.
3. As the rope falls toward your feet rotate your wrists forward to continue the momentum of the rope. Do your two-inch jump just before the rope gets to your feet and use your wrists to keep the rope going under your feet and up over your head again. After you get the rope started, you control the rope with your wrists. Your upper arm, shoulder to elbow, should not be moving much at all.

Exercise Prescription: Jumping Rope

Once you have mastered the skill of jumping rope so that you can jump continuously with only an occasional miss, you can set up an exercise prescription for yourself.

• *Intensity*: Until you are quite expert and efficient at jumping rope, trying to jump at only a moderate pace such as 80 revolutions per minute will probably put your heart rate in your target heart rate zone. You should know that standard jumping rope form calls for one jump per revolution of the rope. With this form 140 revolutions per minute is considered fairly fast and will likely take you to the upper end of your target heart rate zone.

If you are in excellent physical condition and want a jump rope challenge try doing "doubles" for 15 to 30 seconds at a time. A "double" is when the rope goes around your body *twice* for each time you jump. Remember, you control the rope with your wrists. To do doubles, spin the rope faster.

• *Frequency*: As a cross-training alternative you may

only jump rope once or twice a week. If you are a beginner and you wish to master the skill of jumping rope, then you should practice more often.

• *Duration*: With training you will be able to work your way up to 20 minutes of jumping rope, but you can enjoy some cross-training benefits even with shorter workouts. Here is a progressive schedule, which you might find helpful. You can do these workouts once, twice, or three times in a given week, depending on your cross-training needs.

Jump Rope Progression

Week 1: 5 sets of 1:00 each.

Week 2: 5 sets of 1:30

Week 3: 5 sets of 2:00

Week 4: 5 sets of 2:30

Week 5: 5 sets of 3:00

Week 6: 3 sets of 5:00

Week 7: 4 sets of 5:00

Week 8: 2 sets of 10:00

Week 9: 2 sets of 12:00

Week 10: 1 set of 20:00

Rest 10 to 15 seconds between sets.

Cross Training with Rowing Machines

Rowing machines have been in use in the United States since the early 1900s. They first appeared on the East coast where rowing and sculling were popular and competitors needed a way to train during the winter.

A quality rowing machine workout is an excellent cross-training activity for many exercisers and particularly for those whose primary workout is demanding on their legs. A consistent indoor rowing routine can provide you with a well-balanced physical fitness profile. With your weight supported by the seat, the muscular work is divided between your legs, your arms, your shoulders, and your back muscles.

Potential Physical Fitness Benefits Provided by Rowing Machine

Aerobic Capacity	4
Strength Upper Body	4
Strength Lower Body	4
Flexibility Upper Body	3
Flexibility Lower Body	2

These benefits assume the exerciser is following the principles of exercise as described in Chapter 3. Naturally there are some people who will gain more or less than the estimated benefit listed here.

4 = excellent   3 = good   2 = fair   1 = minimal

There are several different types of rowing machines on the market. The T-Bar rower has a single T-Bar rowing arm, foot straps, a seat that rides on one rail, and a hydraulic cylinder that provides resistance.

The dual-action rower has two independent "oars." This type of rower has foot pedals, hydraulic or gas-assisted resistance cylinders, and a padded seat.

The rowing simulators have jointed arms that rotate to simulate the action of actual rowing. Resistance is adjusted by a ratchet and disc-brake mechanism at the joints.

The oarless rower with a flywheel is considered by serious rowers to be the best simulation of real rowing

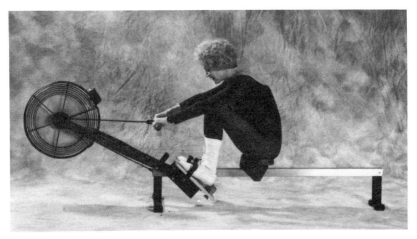

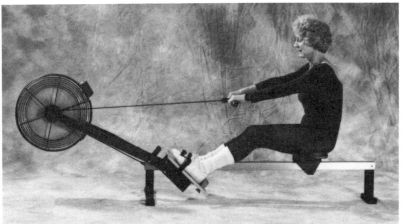

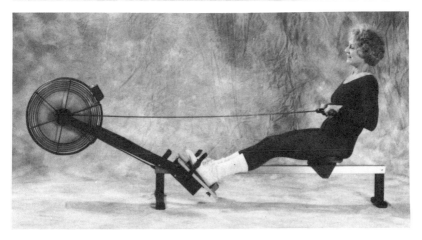

Rowing machine workouts also develop upper body muscle tone and aerobic fitness.

movement. One of the most popular models of oarless rowing machine is the Concept II. It has a seat that slides along a monorail, and in the front of the machine is a flywheel with plastic fins on it. The drive chain wraps around the front wheel and connects to the handle. The Concept II rowers cost close to $700 and the company puts out a terrific newsletter (CII, R.R. 1, Box 1100, Morrisville, VT 05661).

Getting Started: Rowing Machines

Before you begin your workout you need to adjust the foot straps, take a proper grip, and set the resistance for the rear arm lever or handle.

Regardless of the type of mechanism for setting the resistance on your rowing machine, set it low when you are just beginning to row as a cross-training activity. The lower setting will give you a better chance to do a longer, continuous workout. When you can do 20 minutes without stopping it's time to consider increasing the resistance.

Loosen the foot strap from one foot, slide your toes under it and let your heel rest comfortably against the base of your foot pedal.

You may grasp the handle (or lever) overhand or underhand. Don't grip too tightly or your forearms and hands will get tired quickly. During a long workout it may help you to change handgrip positions now and then.

Indoor Rowing Technique

Basic technique is the same for any of the indoor rowing machines.

Step 1: *The Catch*
Start with your knees bent, your body close to the front of the rower, and your upper body leaning slightly forward so that your chest just about touches the front of your thighs.

Step 2: *The Power Stroke*
Push with your feet against the foot pedals. This movement is equivalent to the power stroke in weight lifting so you exhale as you push. As you extend your legs, pull the

handle or rowing arms back with your arm muscles while you are leaning back slightly. Do not lean so far back that your shoulders drop toward the ground. After your legs are fully extended, pull the handle (or rowing arms) smoothly into your chest. Properly done, the power stroke is a fluid motion.

Step 3: *The Recovery*

Push your palms forward and twist your wrists to push the rowing handle (or arms) ahead of your chest. Straighten your arms out and bring your body forward.

Some experienced rowers think of the recovery as though someone is pulling them forward by the hands. First their arms straighten, then the shoulders follow, and finally the upper body leans forward. Once you find yourself in the catch position, you are ready for your next stroke.

Exercise Prescription: Rowing Machines

• *Intensity:* Whether you are doing 5, 20, or 60 minutes of rowing, it is a good idea to check your pulse at least once during your workout to see how your rowing intensity is affecting your heart rate. For maximum cardiovascular fitness benefits you will have to build your upper body so that you are able to work in your target heart zone for 20 minutes continuously. Once your arms, back, and shoulders have this necessary strength and endurance, you can decide whether you want to work harder by increasing the resistance or by pulling faster. Either increase will raise your exercise heart rate and help you burn more calories per workout.

• *Frequency:* As a cross-training alternative you should do your indoor rowing workouts once or twice per week.

• *Duration:* Work your way up to 20 minutes. This can be your standard cross-training workout. You should also know that it is not uncommon for those exercisers who are thoroughly enjoying their indoor rowing or whose goals suggest the need for longer workouts to row for as long as 60 minutes.

Cross Training with Step-Climbing Machines

Step-climbing machines first àppeared on the American exercise scene in the mid-1980s and have since become enormously popular in fitness centers, health clubs, and home gyms throughout the United States. The StairMaster model led the way, but similar machines providing the same type of exercise soon arrived.

Each model of step-climbing machine has its own variations for operation, but the basic movement is the same. You place your feet on large pedals, and as one foot is pressing or moving down, the other foot is going back to the "up" position. You are stepping up and down but the machine stays in the same place.

Step climbing can provide high aerobic fitness and good lower body strength (mainly the front of the thighs because your quadriceps are doing most of the work).

Potential Physical Fitness
Benefits Provided by Step Machine

Aerobic Capacity	4
Strength Upper Body	1
Strength Lower Body	4
Flexibility Upper Body	1
Flexibility Lower Body	2

These benefits assume the exerciser is following the principles of exercise as described in Chapter 3. Naturally there are some people who will gain more or less than the estimated benefit listed here.

4 = excellent   3 = good   2 = fair   1 = minimal

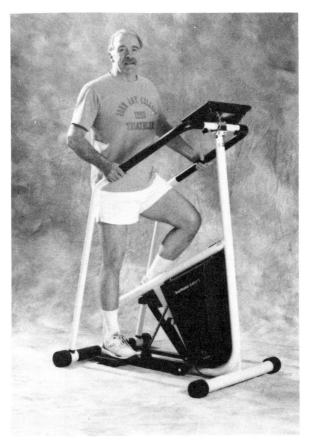

Cross training on a step machine leads to good
aerobic conditioning and outstanding
quadriceps (front of thigh) muscle tone.

Two major reasons exercisers love to do step machine
workouts are the smooth, steady workout they offer, and
the terrific electronic consoles you can program and watch
while stepping. Your body weight is always supported
when you are on the step machine. Your feet never leave
the pedals; you are never airborn the way you are when
running, thus you never have to "land." In other words, a
step machine workout avoids the force of this landing and
the related injuries. Since it is the landing part of running
that is responsible for most of the trauma to the body,
smooth, constant contact movement is easier on the body.
But at the same time the biomechanics of stepping are

close enough to running to provide useful conditioning for runners.

Dr. Steven Loy of the exercise physiology laboratory at Cal State-Northridge found that eight weeks of step training produced results equivalent to eight weeks of outdoor running. Loy recognizes the role cross training plays in many fitness routines. He and other physiologists feel that it may be possible to incorporate step climbing into a running program in a systematic manner.

Many step-climbing machines have colorful console displays to show what you are achieving as you exercise. Many people enjoy this instant feedback. You will be able to see how much time is left in your workout, how many calories you have expended, how far you have traveled in flights of stairs or equivalent mileage, and how many watts you are generating (A watt is a unit of power. Watts and caloric expenditure are discussed in chapter 12, "Work Conversion.") Some step machines even have a program that allows you to give yourself a submaximal cardiovascular fitness test.

The VersaClimber is a variation of the step machine that offers upper body exercise as well. It has no resistance adjustment. You increase the intensity of your workout by stepping faster or higher. The VersaClimber can give you a vigorous workout. Should you find that you are getting tired quickly even at a slow step cadence, try interval training by stepping for two minutes and resting for one. After eight sets you will have completed an excellent total body cardiovascular workout.

Potential Physical Fitness
Benefits Provided by Climbing Machine

Aerobic Capacity	4
Strength Upper Body	4
Strength Lower Body	4
Flexibility Upper Body	3
Flexibility Lower Body	3

These benefits assume the exerciser is following the principles of exercise as described in Chapter 3. Naturally there are some people who will gain more or less than the estimated benefit listed here.

4 = excellent	3 = good	2 = fair	1 = minimal

Form: Step-Climbing Machines

Step climbing is easy. Even so, there are a few pointers to know that will add to the quality of your workout.

- Stand up straight on the pedals. Leaning over or hunching your back are not good for you during a step machine workout.
- Use the handrails for balance, not as support. If you are leaning heavily on the handrails you are doing less work and thereby not getting as much benefit from your workout as you should.
- Follow the instructions provided.
- Stretch your quadriceps and lower back when done.

Exercise Prescription: Step Climbing

- *Intensity*: To improve your cardiovascular fitness and for weight control you should try to work hard enough to bring your heart rate up to your target zone. Most step machines can be programmed at different levels of intensity. Take a conservative approach to your first workout by giving yourself a low level workout. Check your pulse after five minutes and see how your heart rate compares to your target zone. With this information you will be able to adjust your workout accordingly.

• *Frequency:* As a cross-training alternative, step climbing should be done once or twice per week. But, if you are cross training indoors to avoid inclement weather and want to use step climbing to maintain or increase cardiovascular conditioning you would then need to do three or more step climbing workouts per week.

• *Duration:* As for other cardiovascular activities, you should work your way up to 20 minutes continuously. Some models of step-climbing machines have 45-minutes limits on their console programs. If you can do 45 minutes straight you are doing very well.

Programs: The more sophisticated step-climbing machines offer programs that change the pace for you automatically. Your console lights are then displayed in a pattern equal to your workload. Or, you may be on a model that flashes lights at you if you are not keeping up with the pace you programmed. Why all the bells and whistles? To entertain you. To keep you company. To acknowledge your efforts. To allow you to measure your accomplishments.

Note: Interval training can be performed on some step machine models with a manual control feature that allows you to adjust the intensity whenever you like.

Aerobic Cross Training with Treadmills

A treadmill is a machine that has a revolving belt on which you may walk or run while remaining in the same place. Can a treadmill be thought of as a gerbil's exercise wheel redesigned to fit man? Probably. Is a treadmill a terrific machine for aerobic exercise and cross training? Absolutely. Treadmills come in many shapes, sizes, and models. The specifications vary and the type of workout you can do on one treadmill may differ from one model to the next. There are nonmotorized treadmills, which use narrow rollers located under the revolving belt to permit the exerciser to push the belt backward with each stride. The nonmotorized treadmills tend to be less expensive but unfortunately do not provide the same feel to the workout and are far less popular. The moving belt of the motorized treadmill provides a minute mechanical advantage as your foot lands for each stride, though engineers have calculated the effect on the work being done at any given speed as negligible.

If you are able to walk you can enjoy a treadmill workout. You will not need a series of lessons and there is no learning curve. Running smoothly on a treadmill is not hard to do. It may require a couple of sessions, but you are not "learning" so much as you are getting the feel of the moving belt and discovering how to keep your balance.

Both walking and running on treadmills develop aerobic capacity. You should also be aware that many exercisers use treadmills as their primary exercise activity. In either situation, treadmill workouts have advantages you should know about:

- Treadmills are simple to learn
- Moving on a treadmill is easier on your joints than walking or running on pavement. (Most treadmill belts lay on a wooden board which has some give to it.)
- There are no terrain problems such as unsure footing, curbs, mud, etc.
- There is no wind resistance, no rain, no blazing sun, and no freezing cold.
- There are no hills—unless the treadmill has a percent grade feature that allows you to put it on an incline because you want to increase your workload.
- A constant pace can be set. You bring the treadmill up to the speed you want and the belt continues at that speed. By working at this steady pace you are assured of maintaining the speed you need to achieve your exercise goals.
- Partners can exercise side by side even when training at different speeds.
- Many treadmills are equipped with consoles that can be programmed to provide constant information such as: how long you have been on the treadmill; the distance you have traveled; your current pace in miles per hour; and your caloric expenditure.

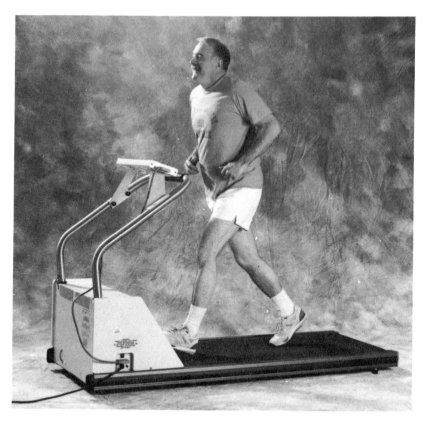

Treadmill workouts enhance aerobic capacity and offer certain advantages over outdoor running such as pace information, comfortable temperature and a level running surface.

Getting Started: Treadmills

Treadmills are available for cross training in commercial exercise facilities, hotel health clubs, Y's, university fitness centers, corporate wellness programs, and homes. If you are going to join a commercial exercise facility remember to ask a few questions before putting up any money (see page 000 for guidelines to selecting a commercial exercise facility).

If you are thinking about purchasing a motorized treadmill for home use these are some questions to consider:

- Does it operate on a 110 outlet?
- How much space will it need?

- Will you be happy doing your workouts without any visual or auditory stimulation? In other words, do you think you might like to watch television or listen to your stereo while exercising on your treadmill? If so, plan placement of the treadmill accordingly. Of course, you can always use headphones if you cannot put the treadmill in the room with the stereo.
- What warranty does your treadmill have?
- What should you expect to spend?

There are several home-use treadmills that go up to six miles per hour (a ten-minute mile) available for close to $1,000. If your exercise goals call for you to run faster, you may have to spend more. But, if you can estimate the number of workouts you will do per year over the next ten years, then your home treadmill will seem well worth the cost.

Exercise Prescription: Treadmills

- *Intensity*: Walking continuously at a brisk space for twenty minutes was found to provide protection against all factors contributing to early death in the largest study ever done examining the benefits of exercise (Institute of Aerobic Research, Dallas, Texas, 1989). So what if walking briskly on the treadmill (usually about 3.0 to 3.75 miles per hour for most adults) does not put your heart rate into your target heart rate zone. There are two approaches to this situation. The first requires access to a treadmill with a percent grade feature. Begin your workout at your normal walking speed and check your pulse after five minutes. If it is below your target heart rate zone put the grade up to 2 percent, walk for another five minutes, and check your pulse again. Increasing the grade only 2 percent every five minutes, you will soon find the grade that causes you to work hard enough to bring your heart rate into your target zone.

The second approach to the situation in which a brisk walking speed does not take you into your target zone is to be aware that walking continuously at some slightly lower heart rate such as 60 percent of target zone (instead of 70 percent) is still providing health benefits. Compare what your heart and body are doing during your workout to the heart and body of a individual living a completely sedentary lifestyle.

• *Frequency*: As a cross-training alternative you should be doing treadmill workouts once or twice a week.

• *Duration*: Try for twenty minutes of continuous walking or running per workout. If your exercise goals are connected to endurance activities you will want to go longer. If your goals are related to activities that require bursts of speed you should develop an interval training workout in which you alternate running hard and running easy within the same workout. Certain sophisticated treadmill consoles on the market can be programmed so that the treadmill belt changes speed every few minutes as per your instructions. You can concentrate on running and do not have to press the console buttons for each speed change.

• *Progression*: If you are in the initial conditioning stage and can only walk for ten minutes, do that, rest, and do another ten minutes. You can work your way up to twenty continuous minutes. When you are able to do that, you can think about whether you want to jog or run on the treadmill.

There are many serious runners, even those training for marathons, who are doing much of their training on treadmills because, as already mentioned, the treadmill workout is easier on their body, and they do not have to deal with traffic, terrain, or weather. Of course, since these factors are part of road racing, runners should keep outdoor workouts as part of their training program.

Cross Training Cycling and In-Line Skating Keep On Rolling:

The bicycle we know was invented in the mid-1800s. Bicycle racing began around 1868, and the world's most famous bicycle race, the Tour de France, was first held in 1903. There was a surge in adult cycling in the United States in 1974 during the first oil embargo, but many of the bikes sold were not of the quality to keep people interested and active. In the late 1970s bicycle engineering began to meet the needs of prospective cyclists when California Gary Fisher introduced the mountain bike. Today, approximately one of every four bikes sold in America is a mountain bike.

In 1986 the popularity of cycling in the United States rose when cyclist Greg LeMond became the first American to win the Tour de France. LeMond's repeat victories in 1989 and 1990 further contributed to the increase in cycling in the United States. In fact, the number of adults who ride regularly (at least once a week) doubled in the five years from 1985 to 1990, going from 12 million to 25 million cyclists, according to estimates from the Bicycle Institute of America.

Getting Started: Cycling

There are several types of outdoor bicycles to choose from when you are ready. No matter which bike you opt for you will be receiving excellent cardiovascular fitness benefits while developing lower body strength and burning calories. Physiologists estimate that on average cyclists utilize 33 calories to ride a mile. If we assume a modest speed of 10 miles per hour and a thirty-minute ride, then you will expend approximately 165 calories on a five-mile workout.

Potential Physical Fitness
Benefits Provided by Cycling (Outdoors)

Aerobic Capacity	4
Strength Upper Body	3
Strength Lower Body	4
Flexibility Upper Body	3
Flexibility Lower Body	3

These benefits assume the exerciser is following the principles of exercise as described in Chapter 3. Naturally there are some people who will gain more or less than the estimated benefit listed here.

4 = excellent	3 = good	2 = fair	1 = minimal

Cycling places much less stress on your lower body joints than activities that involve running or jumping. Therefore, if your primary activity is running, basketball, volleyball, a racquet sport, or any type of skiing, cycling is an excellent cross-training choice for you.

In Greg LeMond's *Complete Book of Bicycling*, he recommends a racing bike for most people. Your energy is transferred efficiently and the bike itself is flexible in terms of how you use it. It is perfect for short trips as well as touring.

If you know that you will be using your bike primarily to cross train or commute, then consider a mountain bike. You will be sitting up straighter, which makes you more visible to drivers; for modest distances you will probably be more comfortable; and with its thicker tires, you will be safer and have fewer flats.

Mountain bikes are also called all-terrain bikes, or ATBs. You should wear a helmet at all times. Your helmet becomes even more important if you use your mountain bike to do actual off-road riding, because the unpredictability of the terrain greatly increases the possibility of a fall.

Hybrid is another recreational bike, and it's name followed logically from it's development. The Hybrid is heavier and has wider, thicker tires than a racing bike, but it's faster than a mountain bike. Hybrids are not designed for off-road riding.

Tandem bikes—the bicycles built for two—are available as road bikes (thinner tires, faster) and as mountain bikes (including 18 gears to help you handle hills more easily). One advantage to tandem bike workouts is that the two riders can enjoy each other's company throughout the ride. Tandem riding is best for a couple who are not dramatically apart in riding strength, unless the weaker rider is content to let his or her feet spin while the stronger rider sets the pace. Tandem bikes are more expensive than other bikes at entry level, beginning at around $1,200.

Recumbent bikes look different, but they are comfortable and are gradually gaining in popularity. These low-slung bikes have a wide, back-supportive seat set low between the wheels and are now being manufactured by more than a dozen companies in the United States. Stuart John Meyers, publisher of *American Bicyclist*, says "Recumbents are far and away the most comfortable and arguably the safest bikes."

Recumbent handlebars may be located under the seat but you will learn how to steer quickly. What will take some time to master is the pedal technique required to ride your recumbent uphill. You'll need to pedal rapidly in lower gears.

The six-speed ReBike begins at $389 (407-750-1304). For a general introduction to recumbent bikes write to the Recumbent Bicycle Club of America (17650-B6 140th Avenue S.E., Suite 341, Renton, WA 98058.

The Fit

Greg LeMond devotes an entire chapter to fitting a traditional racing bike in *The Complete Book of Bicycling*. The first step is to determine the correct frame size relative to your body, then determine what overall height your bike will be, set the saddle height, adjust your cleats, review your pedaling position, evaluate your upper body extension, measure the correct height of the stem, and finally, size your handlebars. Sound a bit complicated? You're right. And fitting by a formula from a book is tricky, too. Solution? Go to a reputable bike shop and explain your goals. A knowledgeable, conscientious salesperson will be able to take you through all the steps involved in determining a proper bicycle fit. There are even computer programs that print out bike specifications based on your inseam and other torso measurements.

Exercise Prescription for Cycling

Intensity: When you are cycling indoors it will be simple for you to check your pulse to determine whether your heart rate is in your target zone. Since your quadriceps are doing almost all of the work while cycling, you may have to concentrate on maintaining a high rpm (revolutions per minute) to keep your heart rate at the appropriate intensity.

Outdoors your heart rate will fluctuate according to changes in the terrain. Check your pulse only while on smooth level ground. (Look at the timer on your cyclocomputer.) Try to maintain a consistent effort. Pedal downhill if it is safe. Keep your rpm's at a steady rate if possible. Fifty rpm's is the lower end of this variable. Competitive cyclists train at 90 to 110 rpm's because their speed is believed to provide the best efficiency for the effort involved.

Frequency: Once or twice per week.

Direction: Twenty minutes per workout minimum. If you enjoy cycling outdoors, you may find yourself touring for hours at a time.

Progression: From twenty minutes per workout, add five minutes, each week according to your enjoyment, available time and fitness goals. Competitive cycling can be thrilling. Join your local club to learn what its all about.

It can be challenging to find the time for your new workouts. Take a look at Chapter 7 (page 000). Cross Training.

Cross Training with In-Line Skating

In-line skating is often referred to as roller blading because Rollerblade, Inc., developed the first in-line skate. Today there are a half-million people in the United States who own a pair of in-line skates, and it's the fastest growing form of exercise in America. If you ride a bike, ski, or skate on ice for any purpose (figure skating, speed skating, ice hockey, or simple recreational skating) you will find in-line skating to be an excellent supplementary cross-training activity because it works the four-part muscle group on the front of your thighs (the quadriceps) extremely well. Nineteen-year-old speedskater Brian Smith (1993 Junior World All-Round Champion) is one of many athletes cross training with in-line skating.

In-line skates usually have four wheels in a single row on each skate. In-line skating actually feels more like ice skating than roller skating, and for the record, in-line skating is easier than ice skating.

In-line skating will provide you with good cardiovascular fitness benefits, once you are able to skate continuously for five minutes. You will have to do four sets of five minutes with a minimum of rest between sets to achieve these benefits. As with cycling, in-line skating avoids the pounding associated with running and running sports.

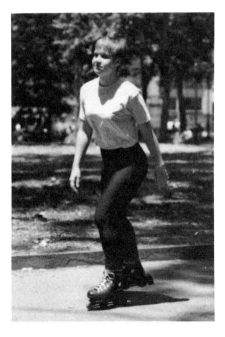

In-line skating is one of the fastest growing forms of exercise in America. Note: For your safety you will want to wear knee pads, elbow pads, wrist guards, and perhaps a helmet too.

Potential Physical Fitness Benefits Provided by In-Line Skating

Aerobic Capacity	4
Strength Upper Body	2
Strength Lower Body	4
Flexibility Upper Body	2
Flexibility Lower Body	3

These benefits assume the exerciser is following the principles of exercise as described in Chapter 3. Naturally there are some people who will gain more or less than the estimated benefit listed here.

4 = excellent	3 = good	2 = fair	1 = minimal

Getting Started: In-Line Skating

Try renting a pair of in-line skates for your first few workouts so that you can evaluate whether you will master in-line skating, and if so, will you be satisfied with the workout it provides? The skates should fit quite snugly, and you should put on wrist guards, knee pads, elbow pads, and a helmet before your first outing. "Fitting" may take twenty minutes. These protective items are usually included with the rental fee. Unless you have a strong skating back-ground you should know that you will probably fall down now and then as you develop your in-line skating skills. If your body is not suited for an occasional fall, take your time and be very careful.

As you head out for your workout there are a few things to keep in mind. Stay on level ground for a while and *practice stopping.* To stop, bend your knees until you are in a crouch position, bring your legs close together, then lift one toe off the ground so the "brake" located on the heel catches the ground and slows you down. Again, practice stopping during the first five minutes of your workout. Mark Powell and John Svensson devote a chapter to brake stops, T-stops, stopping on hills, Y-stops, and hockey stops in their book *In-Line Skating* (Human Kinetics Publishers; 217-351-5076).

Consider limiting your first workout to thirty minutes of skating. You can skate for ten minutes, rest for two or three, and so forth, until you have done thirty minutes altogether. Or, do fifteen minutes, rest, and do fifteen more minutes. Limiting yourself to thirty minutes will keep the soreness your neck and shoulder muscles are likely to feel to a minimum. As with other new activities, once your muscles become accustomed to the tension of the activity you will not feel sore after a workout.

Safety
- - - -

In addition to your protective gear, be aware of your own skating lane. Skaters tend to angle to the left and then back to the right as they push off for each glide.

If you are skating in this manner you must take care that your pushoff does not place you in the path of a bicycle, motorcycle, or vehicle. Listen for warning sounds and look over your shoulder often if you ride in a busy area.

In-Line Skating Purchasing Checklist

- Comfort—Your skates should be comfortable as soon as you lace them up. When you are standing straight your toes should be close to but not touching the front of the boot, and should pull back slightly as you bend your knees.
- Ventilation—The better ventilated your skate the less heat will build up and the more comfortable your feet will be during a good workout.
- Material—The majority of in-line skate boots on the market are made of polyurethane. Serious racers tend to prefer leather. The polyurethane boot is very firm and durable.
- Buckles—Buckles seem to be the trend rather than laces. They are faster to secure and permit you to close your boot with the same tension each time.
- Wheels—If you wear a man's shoe under size 6 or a woman's shoe under size 7 you will usually only need three wheels on your skate. Most skates come with four wheels and some longer frames can accommodate five (which is good for speed but reduces maneuverability).
- Wheels rating Systems—The durometer rating of a wheel ranges from the 70s to the 80s and tells you the degree of hardness of the wheel. The higher the durometer, the softer the wheel. The softer wheel pro-

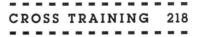

vides a more comfortable ride and more "bite," less slippage on the ground. The harder wheel, a durometer of 78A, for example, is faster.

- Bearings—The bearings are important because they determine how easily your wheels spin. Most bearings are rated 1 to 5, with 5 the fastest.
- Cost—The skates by themselves range from $130 and up, and remember you will need the protective gear mentioned earlier. If you think you will be in-line skating for years to come let your first purchase be a skate with wheels and bearings that can be upgraded easily.

Exercise Prescription: In-Line Skating

- *Intensity*: While you are learning how to do in-line skating do not be overly concerned with your intensity. Presumably, as a beginner, you will have to work fairly hard to master the movements involved. When you find yourself skating for about five minutes without falling or needing to stop, then you can take your pulse and see if it is in your target heart rate zone. If you are working too hard, slow down a little. If you are more than ten beats below the lower end of your target heart rate zone, you may want to try to skate a little harder.
- *Duration*: As mentioned earlier, begin with a thirty-minute workout at the most. To achieve the same calorie expenditure as twenty minutes of jogging, physiologists estimate you would have to do continuous in-line skating for thirty minutes. The mechanical advantage of the skates makes the ratio of jogging to skating roughly 1 to 1.5.
- *Frequency*: Try for once or twice a week. Can you skate for transportation purposes?
- *Progression*: As you skill improves you will be able to skate more efficiently. Eventually you may need to skate longer to feel as though you have done a satisfying workout. There are in-line skaters doing distance workouts of several miles, and there are many skills and stunts to learn if you are so inclined. Racing is an option, too.

Cross Training with Winter Sports: Chill Out

Cross Training with Cross-Country Skiing

Cross-country skiing is a simple and inexpensive sport that is a terrific cross-training option for several reasons. It is easy to learn in one or two lessons, so even beginners get an excellent physical workout. You can ski on beautiful, snowy trails, and you can ski anywhere that there is six inches of snow on the ground. Cross-country skiers are gliding about in the parks of cities such as New York, Chicago, Boston, Montreal, and Detroit. Minneapolis and Toronto have zoos you can visit on skis. Furthermore, you utilize all your major muscle groups in every outing.

Cross-country skiing is a fine family activity as well. Children as young as six can get the motion going and do a beginner's loop of twenty minutes.

Cross-country skiing can be performed by the occasional athlete or by the physical fitness devotee. The two can ski for hours together, with only a slight adjustment on the part of the stronger skier.

In the middle of the 1800s, "Snowshoe Thompson" was doing occupational cross training on skis. Carrying mail along a ninety-mile route across the Sierras gave Thompson an extra measure of endurance work as he became the most famous cross-country skier in the United States.

Getting Started" Cross-Country Skiing

Snow Country magazine periodically discusses the cross-country ski resorts around the country. Excellent equipment is available for modest rental fees and there is a separate fee for getting on the trail. But the most valuable money you will spend on your first day is for a lesson. Your instructor will show you how to glide, when to use the poles, how to stop, turn, and conquer hills, and how to get up when you fall.

Potential Physical Fitness
Benefits Provided by Cross-Country Skiing

Aerobic Capacity	4
Strength Upper Body	4
Strength Lower Body	4
Flexibility Upper Body	4
Flexibility Lower Body	4

These benefits assume the exerciser is following the principles of exercise as described in Chapter 3. Naturally there are some people who will gain more or less than the estimated benefit listed here.

4 = excellent   3 = good   2 = fair   1 = minimal

If you can ski near home on a snowed-over golf course, a hiking trail, a bridle path, a logging road, or some other public land, you may decide it is worthwhile to purchase an introductory package of ski equipment.

Developments in petrochemical technology have led to improvements in cross-country skis. Beginning skiers will usually purchase touring skis because they are wide and stable—they can be used on machine-groomed tracks or wilderness trails. Most touring skis have polyethylene (P-Tex) plastic running surfaces, and the waxless models are patterned underfoot to grip the snow without having to apply wax. The waxless skis have backward slanting protuberances, which allow the ski to slide forward but not back.

Another feature most touring skis have is sidecut. Sidecut is the difference in width between tip, waist, and tail that gives the ski a slight hourglass appearance and makes it easier to turn.

Camber is the amount of flex in the base of the ski. If

you were to press together the bases of a few sets of different kinds of skis, you would get a feeling of how camber stiffness varies among skis.

When you press down on the midsection of a cross-country ski, the camber flattens out and the base comes into contact with the snow. If the base is smooth you will need to apply wax to allow the ski to grip the snow. If the base has a pattern implanted into the plastic running surface it is a waxless ski (described above).

You can ski comfortably in clothes you use for other winter activities. If you find that you want to ski regularly you will appreciate wearing clothes specific to cross-country skiing. For example, hydrophobic polypropylene underwear feels better than it reads and is a good choice for your first layer of clothing—the layer closest to your body. A light wool turtleneck makes a good second layer because it holds warm air close to the body. Your third layer could be a down vest if you usually ski at a slow-to-moderate speed need extra insulation. Your last layer might be a one-piece bib knicker or a two-piece knicker suit made of a comfortable wind-resistant fabric.

Of course, you should have two pairs of socks, a woolen hat, mask or earmuffs, sunglasses or snow goggles, and winter gloves.

Cross-country skiing is clearly one of the most complete forms of exercise and therefore rates high as a cross-training option that offers excellent overall conditioning. In contrast with downhill skiing, cross-country skiing is continuous and thus provides an excellent aerobic workout. In fact, among top athletes, cross-country skiers have been found to have the highest maximal oxygen capacity (also referred to as VO2 MAX). This may be due to the work the upper body muscles do as they pull and push with the ski poles.

While you are developing your physical fitness you will also be improving your balance and concentration, because cross-country skiing involves performing a variety of maneuvers.

Exercise Prescription: Cross-Country Skiing

• *Intensity*: As a learner you need not worry about target heart rate. Once you can ski continuously, which may well be after a one-hour lesson, your heart rate will probably stay in your target heart rate zone during most of your workout—with the time spent getting up from an occasional fall being the cause of a drop in heart rate below target zone.

• *Frequency*: Since you need snow, space, equipment, and time, the frequency of your cross-country skiing workouts will vary according to those factors.

• *Duration*: For your first day out plan to take a one-hour lesson. After that you can go on a beginner trail for 20 to 45 minutes, depending on your endurance. As your skill and conditioning improve you may want to ski for as much as two hours. Many cross-country skiers make a day of it by resting and refueling with a lunch break and then heading back to their starting point afterward.

• *Progression*: After you are able to do a full day of skiing the next challenge can be how far can you go in one day?

Cross Training with Snowboarding

Snowboarding is a new and exciting winter activity in which the athlete slaloms down a slope while standing sideways on a board that resembles a cross between a skateboard and a ski. Snowboarders use bootstraps but not ski poles.

In the past two years snowboarding has grown to a $250 million industry and according to the National Sporting Goods Association, in 1991 there were 1.6 million snowboarders in America.

Getting Started: Snowboarding

"Shredding," as snowboarding is known to its participants, is a lot of fun, but it can be difficult to learn. Dr. Peter Janes, an orthopedic surgeon at Vail Orthopedic and Sports Medicine in Vail, Colorado, recommends lessons and properly fitted equipment for the novice snowboarder. A study conducted at the Rochester Institute of Technology in New York showed that the rate of injury for snowboarding is only three injuries per 1,000 snowboard days—the same as alpine skiing.

Snowboarding gives your quadriceps an excellent workout—once you are shredding more than you are falling. As you are able to stay up longer you will get a better cardiovascular workout, but snowboarding is not an activity in which your heart rate will stay in target zone for twenty minutes straight. Its action is much like downhill skiing, and you will get breaks between runs. Snowboarding's greatest appeal as a cross-training option is the variety, challenge, and excitement it provides.

Potential Physical Fitness Benefits Provided by Snowboarding

Aerobic Capacity	3
Strength Upper Body	1
Strength Lower Body	3
Flexibility Upper Body	1
Flexibility Lower Body	2

These benefits assume the exerciser is following the principles of exercise as described in Chapter 3. Naturally there are some people who will gain more or less than the estimated benefit listed here.

4 = excellent	3 = good	2 = fair	1 = minimal

Exercise Prescription: Snowboarding

• *Intensity*: At first your focus should be on technique not on heart rate. When you can snowboard smoothly to the bottom of the slope, you can check your pulse. If your heart rate is in your target zone you are getting cardiovascular benefits for however long the ride down took. As you become more skilled you will be able to do the same run more efficiently and probably with a lower heart rate.

• *Duration*: Begin with short sessions of an hour or so

(including time spent getting back to the top of the slope). As your balance improves you will be snowboarding more, falling less, and enjoying a better workout.

• *Progression*: The basic goal of progression is to snowboard to the bottom of the slope remaining throughout in a vertical position. Subsequent goals may include snowboarding down longer slopes, steeper slopes, and jumping over obstacles.

Cross Training with Dance: Dance To Your Heart's Content

Your heart will be content, and healthier, too, if you are cross training with dance. The music, the camaraderie, and the smiling make dance a magic form of exercise. Even the most ardent runner will probably admit that for sheer fun a good dance class is even better than a good run. This is not to discount the inner satisfaction provided by a good run, but there is a difference between the dazzling spontaneity of dance and the rhythmic pounding of running.

Dancing is a wonderful cross-training alternative for men and women. If you look at registration figures for aerobic dance, ballet, step, and tap classes you will see there are still more women signed up than men. However, more and more men are enjoying dance classes. They like the diversion from their regular routines. Football players take dance classes to develop their agility and find the classes challenging and stimulating. Serious dancers and knowledgeable fitness professionals have long known that the top male ballet dancers, such as Mikhail Baryshnikov and his contemporaries, are physically on a par with any athlete in the world. And if you think about a full-fledged tap routine, you will realize that these performers have exceptional aerobic and muscular endurance.

History of Aerobic Dance

Since aerobic exercise is continuous in nature and is performed at such an intensity, the oxygen needs of the muscles are met throughout the workout. In an aerobic

dance workout the movements are supposed to be continuous (although you are allowed to stop as needed) and
somewhat rhythmic, according to the beat of the music.

In Jackie Sorenson's *Aerobic Lifestyle Book* (Poseidon
Press, 1983), she points out that in 1971 jogging was not yet
popular and aerobic exercise opportunities for women
were limited. These circumstances led Ms. Sorenson to
develop aerobic dancing, a program that originally ca-
tered almost exclusively to women who were physically
inactive and who wanted an effective way to shape up
that would also be fun. Since then hundreds of thousands
of women and men have taken aerobic dance classes all
over the country.

Late in the 1970s Jane Fonda contributed to the increasing popularity of aerobic dance as she put aerobic
dance routines on videotape. She wrote her first workout
book in 1981 (Simon and Schuster) and has remained
active in promoting exercise.

Sorenson and Fonda both recommended that their
followers consider jogging once or twice a week along with
their aerobic dance workouts. In effect, they were promoting cross training ten years ago!

Aerobic dance is actually a dance potpourri. It offers
ballet, boogie, disco, folk dance, and jazz all rolled into one.

Physical Fitness Benefits of Aerobic Dance

The physical fitness benefits of aerobic dance classes vary
according to the pace of the class, the frequency of arm
movements, whether the class is high impact or low impact, the length of the aerobic segment of the class, and
the instructor's overall style.

Potential Physical Fitness
Benefits Provided by Aerobic Dance
(High Impact)

Aerobic Capacity	4
Strength Upper Body	2
Strength Lower Body	4
Flexibility Upper Body	3
Flexibility Lower Body	4

These benefits assume the exerciser is following the principles of exercise as described in Chapter 3. Naturally there are some people who will gain more or less than the estimated benefit listed here.

4 = excellent   3 = good   2 = fair   1 = minimal

Potential Physical Fitness
Benefits Provided by Aerobic Dance
(Low Impact)

- -

Aerobic Capacity	4
Strength Upper Body	2
Strength Lower Body	3
Flexibility Upper Body	3
Flexibility Lower Body	4

These benefits assume the exerciser is following the principles of exercise as described in Chapter 3. Naturally there are some people who will gain more or less than the estimated benefit listed here.

4 = excellent   3 = good   2 = fair   1 = minimal

Aerobic dance classes can be conducted with music playing at 110 beats per minute (considered a moderate pace) or as fast as 160 beats per minute. Normally, participants keeping up with the 160-beat-per-minute class will be giving their hearts a more vigorous workout than those doing a class conducted at a slower pace.

If the instructor includes frequent, vigorous arm movements the exercise heart rate will be higher and there will be better development of upper body muscle tone and flexibility.

Low-impact aerobic dance is a style of class where one foot is on the ground at all times. Low impact classes are considered easier on the body. Since there is no jumping the intensity level is lower than that of a high-impact aerobic dance class, and it follows that the cardiovascular conditioning benefits of the low-impact class will be somewhat less.

Aerobic dance classes can last anywhere from thirty to

sixty minutes. A typical class will include a warm-up, a main segment of aerobic activity, calisthenics for muscle tone, stretching, and a cooldown. The longer the aerobic segment the more calories expended and the greater the weight control benefits.

In addition to gaining physical fitness benefits, when you take an aerobic dance class you are working on your balance, your agility, and your coordination. When you learn the steps and combinations you feel a sense of accomplishment.

From a cross-training perspective, aerobic dance is a wonderful change of pace from a solitary activity or any competitive sport. You enjoy a well balanced workout that employs your muscles differently than the way they are utilized in your primary activity. You are enjoying conditioning benefits while avoiding overuse injuries when you add an aerobic dance workout to your training schedule.

Getting Started: Aerobic Dance

To cross train with aerobic dance you will need to sign up for a class. To find one call your local health club, college physical education department, dance studio, or other similar recreational fitness organization.

While there are colorful tights and bodysuits available for aerobic dance classes, those outfits are not a requirement by any means. In an average beginner's class you will see all kinds of exercise outfits. If you are self-conscious about your physique wear sweat pants or a big, loose-fitting tee-shirt.

The footwear you choose is important. A quality running shoe will likely provide the needed cushioning. There are exercise shoes advertised as being specifically for aerobic dance. Or, you could purchase a cross-training athletic shoe—several excellent models are now available.

Step Classes are aerobic dance with steps provided to allow a variety of additional choreographed movements. They are fun and provide an excellent workout. In a way step classes are easier for a nondancer because your movements are "hidden" behind your step.

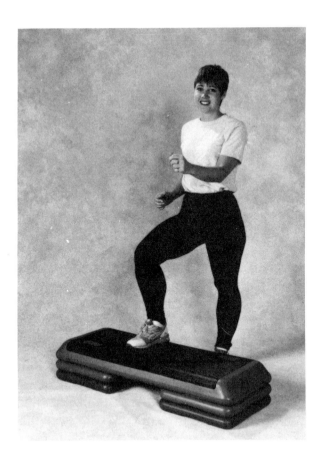

A step workout can be fun with or without the class. At home use a step class videotape and follow the instructor's lead.

Your step can range from 4" to 12" in height. The more fit you are the higher step you will use. After a few simple side to side steps the instructor will have you stepping up and down on the bench, in time with the beat of the music, and you will copy her maneuvers (as best you can).

Each time you step up you are lifting your bodyweight with your legs thus utilizing many large lower body muscle groups. The complete step class will include a brief stretching warm-up. Twenty or more minutes of stepping to provide aerobic exercise benefits (you can always stop and rest if necessary), light hand-weight work for upper body muscle tone, abdominal exercise, more stretching, and a cooldown. The prescription for step class and aerobic dance class is as follows.

Potential Physical Fitness
Benefits Provided by Step Class

Aerobic Capacity	4
Strength Upper Body	2
Strength Lower Body	4
Flexibility Upper Body	3
Flexibility Lower Body	4

These benefits assume the exerciser is following the principles of exercise as described in Chapter 3. Naturally there are some people who will gain more or less than the estimated benefit listed here.

4 = excellent   3 = good   2 = fair   1 = minimal

Exercise Prescription: Aerobic Dance

• *Intensity*: Begin with a low-impact class if possible. For the first few classes don't work too hard. If your instructor has the class checking heart rates you will know if you are exercising in your target zone, but don't worry if you are below target zone while you are getting the feel of the class. When you are keeping up with the combinations a little better you will naturally find yourself getting a better workout.

• *Frequency*: As a cross-training option aerobic dance is excellent for you if done once or twice a week.

• *Duration*: Including the warm-up, aerobic phase, calisthenics, stretching, and a cooldown, the typical aerobic dance class will usually last 45 to 60 minutes.

• *Progression*: If you are in a low-impact class and feel you are not getting enough of a workout, you might want to try a regular class. With some jumping, a faster pace, and a motivational instructor you will soon be enjoying a vigorous workout.

Cross Training with Ballet

Ballet is theatrical entertainment in which ideas are expressed through dancing to musical accompaniment with costumes, scenery, and lighting. Ballet is also a form of dance exercise that requires precise movements. There is one correct way to do First Position—or any other position in ballet. Either your leg is properly stretched, or it is not.

It is this very emphasis on exact positioning that adds to the attractiveness of ballet as a cross-training option. While you are in class you know you must try to move just as your teacher does and to do this you must concentrate. Your head must be up, your shoulders down, your back straight, your stomach in, and your buttocks tucked under your hips. So, not only does ballet provide lower body flexibility and muscle tone, it offers a wonderful mental challenge.

A look at history of ballet enhances any appreciation of the reason each movement must be done just so.

There is no specific moment in the history of dance when ballet can be said to have first appeared. In a sense every dance development, from the first rhythmic movements of primitive man to the accompaniment of the clapping of hands to the stately minuet, was a step leading toward the emergence of the ballet form.

If you are considering adding ballet as a weekly cross-training activity but have not studied ballet before, you should expect to find any class, even a beginner's, challenging. Within a few classes you will have a sense of what you are doing and may well find yourself practicing at home to show your teacher you are improving.

You are likely to discover that one of the best benefits of ballet as a cross-training alternative is its diversity. Ballet is truly different than any other activity (a floor exercise routine in gymnastics comes closest, although the methods of training for floor exercise and ballet differ substantially). No other sport is as demanding when it comes to the precision of the five positions. There are proper mechanics for serving a tennis ball, for example, but if you are getting John McEnroe results you can use an unorthodox serving technique. In ballet there is only one way to do first position—period.

As the following chart shows, ballet provides excellent lower body strength and flexibility. Along with the other physical fitness benefits, your posture is likely to improve when you cross train with ballet.

Potential Physical Fitness Benefits Provided by Ballet (Men)

Aerobic Capacity	3
Strength Upper Body	4 (men do lifts)
Strength Lower Body	4
Flexibility Upper Body	4
Flexibility Lower Body	4

These benefits assume the exerciser is following the principles of exercise as described in Chapter 3. Naturally there are some people who will gain more or less than the estimated benefit listed here.

4 = excellent   3 = good   2 = fair   1 = minimal

Potential Physical Fitness
Benefits Provided by Ballet (Women)

Aerobic Capacity	3
Strength Upper Body	2
Strength Lower Body	4
Flexibility Upper Body	4
Flexibility Lower Body	4

These benefits assume the exerciser is following the principles of exercise as described in Chapter 3. Naturally there are some people who will gain more or less than the estimated benefit listed here.

4 = excellent   3 = good   2 = fair   1 = minimal

Gymnasts who compete in floor exercise events take ballet to increase their grace. Divers cross train with ballet because they find it requires them to be keenly aware of body position at all times. Exercise done in ballet class, such as toe pointing and spotting (looking at a spot on the wall, pivoting your body, swiveling your head quickly until you see the spot again), are relevant to the demands of diving.

Getting Started: Ballet

Find a beginner's class, sometimes called "Adult Ballet," and before registering speak to the teacher to find out whether previous ballet training is expected of the students in the class. Women traditionally wear leotards. They may wear leg warmers and a cutoff tee-shirt, too. A man taking class for the first time would need only a tee-shirt, shorts or sweat pants, and socks. (Ballet shoes are not usually required for a beginner's class.) If you find you like the ballet workout enough to attend consistently you can invest in contemporary ballet attire.

It is a good idea to arrive in the dance studio fifteen to twenty minutes before the class is scheduled to begin so you can do your own stretching routine and warm your muscles.

Follow the teacher's instructions the best you can—there is a great deal to learn and you will not master it all in one class. For example, you will need to listen carefully as the teacher announces the name of each movement since almost all the terms in ballet are French. As in other activities that engage muscles in unfamiliar movements, an expected outcome in a certain amount of muscular soreness 24 to 48 hours after the workout.

As always, listen to your body. If your hips socket is not ready to rotate out the way the teacher would like, just do the best you can—with time you will improve.

Exercise Prescription: Ballet

• *Intensity*: The majority of a beginner's ballet class is spent doing various precise movements over and over again (eight counts and sixteen counts are used often). Your legs work hard but not continuously so your heart rate will be above resting but probably not in your target heart rate zone for most of the class. If the teacher asks you to do jetés (jumps) or another comparable movement then your heart rate will go up into your target zone.

• *Frequency*: Although progress will be slow, cross-training athletes without ballet background will be well served by one class per week for the first eight weeks or so.

• *Duration*: A beginner's ballet class usually lasts sixty minutes.

• *Progression*: You will learn more and move better with every class you take.

Cross Training with Folk Dance

Every country in the world has its own traditional dances. These folk dances are recreational dances performed for pleasure. When you are folk dancing you may not be thinking of it as exercise, but if you are doing another activity consistently and folk dancing weekly, you will be cross training and receiving the many benefits that come with cross training, including meeting new friends, avoiding boredom, and better physical fitness.

When it comes to American folk dance it is fortunate that the Pilgrims did not have the final say. As late as 1850, the Reverend Jesse Guernsey of Derby, Connecticut, was preaching against the evils of dance, which he called "the source of vast mischief." The reality is that folk dancing is the source of vast enjoyment for members of many clubs and organizations, whether religious in nature or not.

Folk dances in America still known by their national names are the Irish jig, the Highland Fling (Scottish), the Italian tarantella, La Cucaracha (Mexico), the Israeli *hora*, and the calypso dances from the Caribbean. From an exercise viewpoint, the cossack step called the *prysiadka* places Ukrainian folk dancing among the most vigorous in the world. You may remember seeing this difficult Ukrainian step where men bend their knees and, in a squatting position, kick out their legs in front of them. (This is hard on the knee joint and is not recommended for everyone.)

Folk dance is characterized by the fact that it exists for the enjoyment of the participants and not for the entertainment of the onlooker. It's a fine cross-training option because it can be danced outdoors in a garden, in a barn, in a nightclub, in a gym, or a tent.

Getting Started: Folk Dance

The many folk dances differ greatly, yet they can be grouped together for an analysis of potential physical fitness benefits. Fortunately, most folk dances have similar physical characteristics: Legs are used for movement whether backpedaling, hopping, jumping, shuffling, skipping, or stepping. During folk dancing the chest and arms are not usually utilized in such a way as to develop strength significantly.

Working from these two analyses, it is fair to say that folk dance generally provides moderate to excellent aerobic benefits and no or little development of the upper body. The physical fitness benefits of folk dance can vary from one dance to another. In the Irish jig, for example, the torso is held very straight with the arms hanging at the side, and it rates low for offering upper body benefits. But the Irish jig dancer can tap as many as three hundred taps per minute—giving it a high rating for providing lower body muscular endurance. With a little thought you can probably come up with a good analysis of the specific physical fitness benefits of your favorite folk dance.

Potential Physical Fitness Benefits Provided By Folk Dance

Aerobic Capacity	3
Strength Upper Body	2
Strength Lower Body	3
Flexibility Upper Body	2
Flexibility Lower Body	2

These benefits assume the exerciser is following the principles of exercise as described in Chapter 3. Naturally there are some people who will gain more or less than the estimated benefit listed here.

4 = excellent	3 = good	2 = fair	1 = minimal

Many churches and community oriented organizations have weekly dances. A few phone calls will get you the details of an upcoming event.

Exercise Prescription: Folk Dance

• *Intensity*: Keep up with the pace of the dancing the best you can. If you meet someone cute and you would like to have a little extra physical contact, ask if he or she would take your pulse for you. This request will lead you to provide an explanation of target heart rate and the benefits of cross training—and who knows what else . . .

• *Duration*: Folk dancing is usually a social event that

last for hours. You dance, socialize, have refreshments, dance some more. To take advantage of cross-training fitness benefits of folk dance, you will be better off spending more time dancing and less time devouring the food.

- *Frequency*: Once or twice per week seems appropriate.
- *Progression*: With practice, your folk dancing skill and stamina will improve.

Cross Training Outdoors:
Going Wild In The Wilderness

The four activities below are enjoyed outdoors and, at first glance, might appear to be out of the realm of "training" as it is generally defined for physical fitness and sporting purposes. However, closer study lets us easily see that each of these activities involves a great deal of movement by large muscle groups for extended periods of time. Aerobic, muscular, and flexibility conditioning are taking place when you add any of these forms of outdoor exercise to your training.

Backpacking takes you on scenic trails and lets you exercise comfortably as you walk through nature's wonder. Canoeing and rowing are performed recreationally and as serious competitive sports. Orienteering, the art of navigation through an unknown area, is a sport that requires problem solving and running. Rock climbing can be done safely and offers excellent strength and endurance benefits. Each of these activities can be enjoyed without any element of competition. You set your own goals, you set your own pace, and you are able to immerse yourself in the activity without concern for some outside standard of performance.

Cross Training with Backpacking

Backpacking is lots of walking with a pack on your back and a pure feeling of independence. A short hike on level ground is a good way to enjoy a first taste of backpacking. A day hike can be done in a state park that has a trail system for hikers. If you progress to overnight backpacking your trip will be accented by areas that offer everything you would expect in the wilderness: great mountain views and beautiful woods, wildflowers, meadows, and ponds.

Hippocrates once said "Walking is man's best medicine." Though I say, "Exercise is our best preventive medicine," the message is clear in either case.

An experienced backpacker may be able to walk fifteen to twenty miles in a day. Excellent lower body muscular endurance is the primary requirement for such a trek, hence backpacking's high rating on the Physical Fitness Benefits chart below. If you stay at a walking pace and do not have to negotiate steep hills, backpacking will provide you with moderate benefits for the other components of physical fitness as well.

Potential Physical Fitness Benefits Provided By Backpacking

Aerobic Capacity	3
Strength Upper Body	3
Strength Lower Body	3
Flexibility Upper Body	1
Flexibility Lower Body	3

These benefits assume the exerciser is following the principles of exercise as described in Chapter 3. Naturally there are some people who will gain more or less than the estimated benefit listed here.

4 = excellent	3 = good	2 = fair	1 = minimal

Getting Started: Backpacking

You will need comfortable, sturdy hiking shoes (sneakers will do on a smooth trail), appropriate clothing, food, your backpack, some camping gear (see list), and a healthy respect for nature.

Consider taking a class on the fundamentals of backpacking. It will likely be followed by a trip. Or, you could join a regional or national outdoor organization such as the Appalachian Trail Conference, the Sierra Club, or the Wilderness Society.

Let your first hike be a pleasant experience so you will want to do again. Until you have some backpacking experience it's a good idea to stay on or close to a trail. Before you go off the beaten path you should know how to use a compass and handle a topographic map.

Overnight Backpacking Camp Gear List

Backpacker's stove	Toilet paper	First-aid kit
Lightweight mess kit	Towel	Flashlight
Cup, spoon, pocket knife	Bug spray	Map
Ground cloth	Sunscreen	Waterproof matches
Foam sleeping pad	Sunglasses	Rope
Lightweight sleeping bag	Biodegradable soap	Water bottle
Rain gear	Compass	Trash bag

Exercise Prescription: Backpacking

• *Intensity:* Walk at the pace you find comfortable. Stop and rest as you feel the need. You do not need to check your pulse, although there is no harm in doing so.

• *Duration:* You can go on for two hours, two days, or two weeks, depending on your readiness.

• *Progression:* If you walk farther in each outing you will eventually enjoy more time in the wilderness.

Cross Training with Canoeing

You can learn to canoe, and you may well find you're glad you did. The canoe makes larger a world that is becoming smaller. "Adventure is where you find it," says Dave Harrison in *Canoeing: Skills for the Serious Paddler*, "and only time and appetite should limit the extent of one's journey."

Canoeing can be done for the simple pleasure of a weekend paddle or for the excellent exercise benefits. It is both an activity in itself and a means to the enjoyment of other pursuits. The canoe is often the method of transport for artists, athletes, birdwatchers, fisherman, geologists, historians, photographers, and prospectors. When you are paddling your graceful, quiet canoe over the water you may find yourself assuming more than one of these roles.

The canoe of the Algonquin Indian has been improved only slightly over the years, and the improvements have been in the materials used, not in the shape of the hull. The canoe combines beautifully the elements of speed, maneuverability, lightness, and carrying capacity.

During portage, when the canoe is carried over land, upper body cross training occurs. At the end of the nineteenth century, Henry Rushtin's 18.5-pound Nessmuk model made canoe portage possible over greater distances. Today canoes are made of aluminum, wood, fiberglass, Kevlar, polyethylene, vinyl, and ABS (acrylonitrile-butadiene-styrene). Designs include flat bottom, round bottom, deep V, shallow V, straight keel, moderate rocker, and high rocker.

The uses of canoes vary widely. Will you be using yours for pleasure, family outings, trips, flat-water racing, or white-water racing? Your answer to this question will help guide you to the right canoe should you decide you are ready for purchase.

Potential Physical Fitness
Benefits Provided By Canoeing

Aerobic Capacity	4
Strength Upper Body	4
Strength Lower Body	1
Flexibility Upper Body	4
Flexibility Lower Body	1

These benefits assume the exerciser is following the principles of exercise as described in Chapter 3. Naturally there are some people who will gain more or less than the estimated benefit listed here.

4 = excellent   3 = good   2 = fair   1 = minimal

Physical Fitness Benefits of Canoeing

As the Chart above shows, canoeing rates well for developing aerobic capacity and upper body fitness.

If you can canoe only a few times a year you may find yourself experiencing fitness benefits and muscular soreness in equal doses, unless you do a short outing. For a better workout and to keep the soreness in check you would be well advised to do at least six weeks of upper body strength training in preparation for canoeing (see chapter 5, "Cross Training for Strength," for specific exercises).

Canoe "marathons" are races that range from five to ten to thirty miles, and ultra-marathons can be several hundred miles and last a few days. Most of the marathon races are organized to attract the citizen (amateur) racer, and many classes are geared toward recreational hulls. If you are able to canoe two or three or more times per week in preparation for a canoe marathon you can expect significant physical fitness benefits.

Getting Started: Canoeing

If your circumstances permit you to purchase a canoe, you are off to a great start. You will be choosing the best craft for you (and your family) according to where you live, how you vacation, how often you expect to canoe, and the type of available water. Regarding price, buy the best canoe you can afford.

You'll need paddles, life preservers, sturdy line (bow and stern line are called painters), a sponge, and a bailer.

To carry the canoe along you will need a carrying yoke.

If you will be canoeing for extended periods of time, your knees will hold up better if you install knee pads in the bottom of the canoe.

Duct tape, also referred to as "boat tape," can patch small or large cracks, a torn rain coat, or a broken cooler. It can protect a paddle shaft from constant contact with the gunwale and has many uses besides patching and protecting. Take a roll with you.

You will need a waterproof bag of some type. The perfect combination of accessibility, durability, and water-tightness will be discovered one day. In the meantime consider what size waterproof bag you need, what weight you are willing to carry, durability, and whether you can open and close it easily. Dedicated canoers search for the perfect waterproof bag the way skiers and swimmers search for "fog-free" goggles.

Exercise Prescription: Canoeing

For recreational canoeing, you paddle as hard as you wish and rest when necessary. If you do a particular route you can time yourself and set training goals to work toward as your technique and endurance improve.

- *Frequency:* Get out on the water as often as circumstances permit. If you are fortunate enough to be able to canoe daily for a few weeks or more, listen to your body for signs telling you to take a day off. Unusual soreness or general fatigue are indicators to skip a day of canoeing.
- *Duration:* The duration of your outing should be appropriate to your stamina. It's better to do a short trip (45 minutes on calm water) the first time out and enjoy it than

to do too much and end up cursing canoeing as an outdated mode of water transportation.

• *Progression:* As your endurance and knowledge of canoeing increase, you may wish to try longer trips or more challenging waterways.

"Cunning Running": Cross Training with Orienteering

Orienteering is the art of navigation through an unknown area using a map and compass as guide. It is a useful survival skill for anyone involved in outdoor activities that take place far from the traveled highways of civilization. Orienteering is a fascinating cross-training option because it combines measurements, calculations, and exercise into one fitness-enhancing activity.

Orienteering began in the United States in 1946 when Bjorn Kjellstrom of Sweden organized a demonstration meet in the Indiana Dunes State Park. In the mid-1960s Norwegian orienteer Harold Wibye initiated a new push for orienteering in the Delaware Valley area. At about the same time, the United States Marine Corps Physical Fitness Academy in Quantico, Virginia, became aware of the sport and initiated a program on orienteering for the Marines. Interest in the new sport then picked up among other branches of the armed forces, especially the army. Its Reserve Officer Training Corps units were soon active in orienteering at many American colleges and universities, helping to make the sport more widely known.

Potential Physical Fitness
Benefits Provided By Orienteering

Aerobic Capacity	4	(in competition)
Strength Upper Body	2	
Strength Lower Body	4	(in competition)
Flexibility Upper Body	2	
Flexibility Lower Body	2	

These benefits assume the exerciser is following the principles of exercise as described in Chapter 3. Naturally there are some people who will gain more or less than the estimated benefit listed here.

4 = excellent   3 = good   2 = fair   1 = minimal

If you are orienteering for the pleasure and cerebral challenge of the sport and do not plan to push yourself physically you will gain physical fitness benefits comparable to those provided by walking and jogging.

If you like working harder, or if you place yourself in an orienteering competition, the running you do between navigational calculations will develop your aerobic capacity more completely than walking or jogging.

Getting Started: Orienteering

To orienteer all you need is a map, a compass, and suitable outdoor clothing. If you wish to try your hand at orienteering competition you will want to contact an orienteering club.

The clothing needs for orienteering include appropriate footwear, layers on top, long pants that won't snag, and head gear for extreme temperatures.

The footwear choices are hiking boots (warm, dry, provide support but are heavy and therefore slow), running shoes (get a pair with nylon uppers so you can wash them easily), orienteering shoes or "knobbies,"—which are similar to running shoes. They are made of waterproof reinforced nylon with studded soles.

Exercise Prescription: Orienteering

Set your own pace for a time that you can handle comfortably. Go two to four times a month if you can. Consider competing to ensure a hard workout.

Cross Training with Rowing

As with canoeing, your rowing workout will find you gliding rhythmically on a nearly silent conveyance while enjoying the clean environment of air and water.

For the sake of simplicity the terms oars and rowing are used here, although technically the correct term for a pair of oars is sculls and the movement performed with them is sculling.

While there are several sports where the athlete moves in a backward direction—the Fosbury Flop high jump and the back-handsprings in gymnastics come to mind—rowing and the backstroke are the only two Olympic events that are performed entirely backward. By turning your back to the bow of your craft and bracing your feet you are able to use the strength of your legs, arms, and back, thus putting more energy into each stroke and producing more power. There are only a few activities that allow so many muscle groups to be engaged during every repetition. As you can see in the Potential Physical Fitness Benefits Provided By Rowing Chart, rowing is an outstanding cross-training option for developing overall physical fitness.

Potential Physical Fitness
Benefits Provided By Rowing

Aerobic Capacity	4
Strength Upper Body	4
Strength Lower Body	4
Flexibility Upper Body	4
Flexibility Lower Body	3

These benefits assume the exerciser is following the principles of exercise as described in Chapter 3. Naturally there are some people who will gain more or less than the estimated benefit listed here.

4 = excellent   3 = good   2 = fair   1 = minimal

The honor of developing boats for rowing seems to go to the Egyptians. Their boats appear on ancient stone walls from 3000 B.C. These boats were powered by sail and oar, and for centuries slaves were used to pull the oars. The first form of recreational rowing appeared in the early eighteenth century on the Thames. Bargemen of that English river raced their crafts as an outgrowth of their occupation.

In 1852 the first Yale-Harvard Race was staged in boats similar to the English racing boats. In 1870 the Yale oarsmen appeared wearing greased leather pants. This was no attempt to be kinky. Rather, they locked their feet in place and slid back and forth on smooth wooden planks, incorporating the power of their legs into their rowing stroke. A year later, the rolling seat was invented. The racing shell consisted then of a narrow hull, wide outriggers to spread the oarlocks, footblocks to anchor the feet, and a sliding seat.

Changes in the design of the racing shell for the next hundred years consisted of refinements and the introduction of new materials and construction methods, not conceptual innovations.

Then, about twenty years ago a naval architect named Arthur Martin combined the sliding seat and outriggers of the racing shell with an easily driven hull, thus giving birth to a terrific form of exercise—modern recreational rowing.

Getting Started: Rowing

A recreational rowing boat is a modern, sliding-seat pulling boat designed for use in open water by rowers of varying ability. If you plan to buy a boat, there are many factors to consider—type of use, cost, capacity, construction, safety, and appearance.

If your rowing background consists of taking a rented wooden rowboat out on a park lake for an hour or so every other summer, you would benefit greatly from lessons (see "Rowing Skills" below for an idea of how much there is to learn about rowing). Contact a rowing club or a rowboat dealer and get an opportunity to take a few lessons, row some different boats, and learn how to set up your boat for maximum efficiency. Visiting several dealers and going to a boat show will allow you to collect a lot of valuable information about different boat designs.

What do you expect from rowing? Whether you seek solitude on the still water of a glassy lake or family fun, as long as you are dipping those oars and pulling hard you are getting the fitness benefits shown earlier. But, since the boat you choose should match your needs, you will have to compare boats for stability and speed. Speed is fun because it is exciting to move your boat through the water quickly. Stability gives you confidence, and having a seaworthy boat means it is safer—it will handle more easily in rough conditions.

In the language of rowing a "double" has nothing to do with second base. A double is a boat designed for two people to row, and a "standard double" cannot be rowed by a single person. There are doubles that can be converted to a single. There are even triple-seat rowboats. But be sure you will have two rowing partners available on a regular basis before you invest in a triple.

Rowing Skills

Chapters have been written about the skills needed to row effectively, efficiently, and enjoyably. There is much for the novice rower to learn. You must know how to tune and pitch your oarlocks, how to set the buttons on the oars, where to place the foot-stretchers, how to board your boat, how to back and turn—and how to row correctly. Developing a beautiful, fluid, powerful stroke is one of the ongoing lures of this sport, and when you finally feel that your own stroke is improving you will be thrilled.

Go out with a knowledgeable friend or arrange for professional lessons. Learning the skills and techniques of rowing correctly from the beginning will in the long run allow you to enjoy the sport and your workouts much more.

Exercise Prescription: Rowing

• *Intensity*: Row easily for five minutes, then check your pulse. If your heart rate is in your target zone you are getting cardiovascular benefits and you may continue at that intensity. If you are below target zone try to pull harder while maintaining proper form.

• *Frequency*: As for canoeing, get out of the water as often as circumstances permit. If you are able to row daily for several weeks, listen to your body for indications that you need a day of rest.

• *Duration*: Twenty minutes of rowing at target heart rate will give you health benefits. When the weather's right and you feel strong, you will surely want to row longer.

• *Progression*: As your endurance, knowledge, and goals change, you may look for extended workouts.

12

Work Conversion

With all the research that has been done on the human body, there is still much to be discovered about precisely how it works. The processes by which we convert one form of energy, food, into another form of energy, muscular contractions, take place at the cellular level and are not yet fully understood. But without studying biochemistry you can learn much of what we do know about work conversion, work comparison, and energy expenditure of the human organism. Understanding these areas will enable you to do your cross training confident that your new workout options are providing cardiovascular health benefits comparable to your primary workout activity. You will also learn about energy balance and weight control. We will begin with a few definitions:

Aerobic Point System—a fitness program developed by Dr. Ken Cooper that assigns point values for the different types of exercise involved. To develop cardiovascular fitness you are expected to earn thirty "aerobic points" per week.

Basal Metabolic Rate (BMR)—the amount of energy used in a unit of time by a fasting, resting subject to maintain vital functions. The rate, determined by the amount of oxygen used, is expressed in calories consumed per hour per square meter of body surface area or per kilogram of body weight.

Calorie—in this chapter this will refer to the large calorie (Calorie), which is the amount of heat necessary to increase the temperature of one kilogram of water by one degree celsius.

Calorimeter—a device used for measuring quantities of heat generated by friction, by chemical reaction, or by the human body.

Energy—the capacity to do work or to perform vigorous activity. Human energy is usually expressed as muscle contractions and heat production, made possible by the metabolism of food.

Energy Cost of Activities—the metabolic cost in calories of various forms of physical activity.

Heart Rate—the number of times the left ventricle of your heart contracts per minute (see Pulse).

Indirect Calorimetry—the measurement of the amount of heat generated in an oxidation reaction, determined by the intake or consumption of oxygen or by measuring the amount of carbon dioxide (or nitrogen) released and translating these qualities into a heat equivalent.

Lean Body Weight—equal to the weight of the body after fat tissue weight is subtracted.

Met—an abbreviation for Metabolic Equivalent. One MET is equivalent to an oxygen uptake of 3.5 milliliters per kilogram of bodyweight per minute. You can also think of a MET as a multiple of your resting metabolism. Sitting still you are doing one MET worth of work. Walking very slowly you are doing about two METS of work. Walking at 2.6 miles per hour puts you at a three MET workload. Jogging at 6.0 miles per hour means you are working at ten METS.

Oxygen Consumption—the amount of oxygen in millimeters per minute required by the body for normal aerobic metabolism.

Pulse—the regular, recurrent expansion and contraction of an artery produced by waves of pressure caused by the ejection of blood from the left ventricle of the heart as it contracts. Your pulse is easily detected on superficial arteries such as the radial and carotid, and it corresponds to each beat of your heart. The normal number of pulse beats per minute in the average adult varies from 60 to 80, with fluctuations occurring with exercise, injury, illness, and emotional reactions.

Rating of Perceived Exertion (RPE)—a psychophysical scale devised for subjective rating of exercise intensity. The original RPE scale uses a range from six to twenty. The revised scale uses a range from zero to ten.

Spirometer—an instrument that measures and records the volume of inhaled and exhaled air.

Watt—the unit of electric power or work in the meter/kilogram/second system of notation. When you use a machine that gives a readout in watts, you are generating the displayed amount of power at that moment. For example, if you row for ten minutes and average 50 watts per stroke on a Concept II rowing ergometer you generate enough energy to light a 50-watt light bulb. For 1,600 meters (one mile) this workout would result in an energy expenditure of approximately 80 calories.

Work—a force moving through a distance (Work = Force x distance). The metabolic equivalent of work is the total energy expended in performing the mechanical work. A typical unit of energy is a calorie.

The conversions listed below will be useful to you when you are doing calculations necessary to compare workouts. Many exercise machines now offer this information on a computer console.

Conversions

Distance	1 mile = 1.6 kilometers
Weight	1 kilogram = 2.2 pounds
Work	1 liter oxygen (00) = 5 Calories
Power	1 MET = 3.5 ml/kg/min
	1 MET = 1.6 kilometers/hour*
	1 MET = 1.0 miles/hour*

*Running on a horizontal surface

Measuring Energy

The direct measurement of heat production in humans can be accomplished with the use of a chamber known as a human calorimeter, but its use is limited. Caloric and energy expenditure are most often measured by open-circuit spirometry. With a spirometer it is possible to analyze the composition of exhaled air. When this measurement shows less oxygen that means the body is using more oxygen. Oxygen consumption can easily be converted to a value for energy expenditure.

Consuming one liter of oxygen liberates 4.82 calories of heat energy, usually rounded off to 5.0 calories. Knowing that average oxygen consumption at rest is 0.235 liters per minute, we can calculate an average value for energy output per minute: 0.235 liters/minute x 5 cal = 1.18 calories per minute.

Multiplying 1.18 x 1440 (the number of minutes in a day) gives us 1699.2—let's call it 1700. Seventeen hundred calories is an approximate value for daily energy expenditure at rest. Your own resting daily energy expenditure may be lower or higher depending on your overall surface area, your body weight, or your lean body weight. As you may remember from chapter 5, your lean body weight includes muscle tissue that requires far more energy to maintain than fat tissue. This is one of the benefits of strength training as it relates to weight control—increased muscle mass means your energy expenditure is raised, even when you are not exercising.

Using the estimate of 1.18 calories per minute as a typical value for an adult's energy expenditure, we can see how exercise plays a dramatic role in the energy equation. When a 140-pound person goes for a modest-paced jog at 5.0 miles per hour the calorie expenditure jumps to 9.0 calories per minute. In twenty minutes of walking this 140-pound exerciser is now expending 180 calories total, 156 calories more than would have been expended at rest. Four such workouts per week gives an increase in calorie expenditure of 624 calories. With calorie intake constant, this increase in calorie expenditure would result in a one-pound weight loss every five and a half weeks, or over nine pounds per year. If the same individual simultaneously reduced caloric intake by just 50 calories per day, the annual weight loss would project to approximately fourteen pounds. Is weight loss usually this neat and clean? Certainly not, as millions of Americans will tell you. But many of those Americans who have reduced their percentage of bodyfat and stayed at a lower, healthier weight will also say that exercising regularly has been a key.

Comparing Intensity Levels of
Your Cross-Training Workouts

Comparing Workout Intensity by Heart Rate

Intensity is measured most often by checking your pulse. The higher the heart rate during exercise the greater the intensity. When you add a new activity to your exercise program you can easily see how it compares to your primary activity by finding your pulse (as explained in chapter 6).

Comparing Workout Intensity by METs

Using heart rate to compare intensity for noncontinuous activities such as downhill skiing or tennis, for example, can be misleading. If you check your pulse just after a challenging run down the slope or at the end of a long

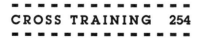

point during which you went from the baseline to the net and back, you will find your heart rate racing. You know that you don't maintain that intensity throughout your workout. For these types of activities you can compare intensity by using MET levels. Use the table on page 256, "Leisure Activities in METs," to compare your primary activity with your new option. Continuing our example, the downhill skier works in the 5–8 MET range and the tennis player works in the 4–9 MET range. Cycling at 10 miles per hour has a MET value of 7 and would be a fine cross-training conditioning option for a downhill skier or tennis player.

Leisure Activities in METs:
Sports, Exercise Classes, Games, Dancing.

	Mean	Range
Archery	3.9	3–4
Back Packing	—	5–11
Badminton	5.8	4–9+
Basketball		
Gameplay	8.3	7–12+
Non-game	—	3–9
Billiards	2.5	—
Bowling	—	2–4
Boxing		
In-ring	13.3	—
Sparring	8.3	—
Canoeing, Rowing and Kayaking	—	3–8
Conditioning Exercise	—	3–8+
Climbing Hills	7.2	5–10+
Cricket	5.2	4.6–7.4
Croquet	3.5	—
Cycling		
Pleasure or to work	—	3–8+
10 mph	7.0	—
Dancing (Social, Square, Tap)	—	3.7–7.4
Dancing (Aerobic)	—	6–9
Fencing	—	6–10+
Field Hockey	8.0	—
Fishing		
from bank	3.7	2–4
wading in stream	—	5–6
Football (Touch)	7.9	6–10
Golf		
Power cart	—	2–3
Walking (carrying bag or pulling cart)	5.1	4–7
Handball	—	8–12+
Hiking (Cross-country)	—	3–7
Horseback Riding		
Galloping	8.2	—

Leisure Activities in METs: Sports, Exercise Classes, Games, Dancing. *(Continued)*

	Mean	Range
Trotting	6.6	—
Walking	2.4	—
Horseshoe Pitching	—	2–3
Hunting (Bow or Gun)		
Small game (walking, carrying light load)	—	3–7
Big game (dragging carcass, walking)	—	3–14
Judo	13.5	—
Mountain Climbing	—	5–10+
Music Playing	—	2–3
Paddleball, Racquetball	9	8–12
Rope Jumping	11	—
60–80 skips/min	9	—
120–140 skips/min	—	11–12
Running		
12 min per mile	8.7	—
11 min per mile	9.4	—
10 min per mile	10.2	—
9 min per mile	11.2	—
8 min per mile	12.5	—
7 min per mile	14.1	—
6 min per mile	16.3	—
Sailing	—	2–5
Scubadiving	—	5–10
Shuffleboard	—	2–3
Skating, Ice and Roller	—	5–8
Skiing, Snow		
Downhill	—	5–8
Crosscountry	—	6–12+
Skiing, Water	—	5–7
Sledding, Tobogganing	—	4–8
Snowshoeing	9.9	7–14
Squash	—	8–12+
Soccer	—	5–12+
Stairclimbing	—	4–8
Swimming	—	4–8+
Table Tennis	4.1	3–5
Tennis	6.5	4–9+
Volleyball	—	3–6

Comparing Workout Intensity by Rating of Perceived Exertion (RPE) scale

You can also evaluate your intensity of exercise subjectively. At some point during your next workout, make a judgment as to how hard you *feel* you are working. Use the Rating of Perceived Exertion scale, (p. 16) which goes from 6 to 20. If you do continuous, steady pace exercise you will find it is a simple matter to judge how hard you are working. You just have to make a mental note to rate your effort during the middle portion of your workout.

If you are playing a stop-start type of game like squash, you could evaluate the entire match. If you won 15–2, 15–4, 15–1, chances are you were not working too hard and wouldn't rate your RPE effort at 18. Your opponent was probably doing most of the running and your RPE for this match might be 11 or so.

If our squash player added jogging to his exercise program, he could ask, "How hard am I willing to work when I cross train?" If satisfied with the aerobic conditioning provided competing at an RPE of 11, the player can make a conscious effort to jog at a pace that feels the same. If he would like a higher level of aerobic fitness to win the club squash tournament, he will need to add faster-pace running to the jogging workouts. During this running he will work at an RPE of 16 to 18—it won't be in the comfort zone, but that's the effort involved if you want a higher level of performance.

Comparing Workouts by the Cooper Aerobic Point System

Many exercisers like to track the quantity of their aerobic workouts with Dr. Ken Cooper's aerobic points. This system can be used to compare the aerobic fitness values of different activities. A full explanation of Dr. Cooper's system can be found in his book, *The Aerobics Program for Total Well-Being* (New York: M. Evans, 1982).

Energy Expenditure and Work Conversion

There are energy expenditure tables available which tell you how many calories you are expending per minute for

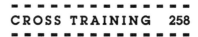

a given activity. With a few simple calculations you can then compare the caloric expenditure of your primary workout with your cross training option.

One of the best energy expenditure tables can be found in Katch and McArdle's text, *Introduction to Nutrition, Exercise and Health*, 4th edition, Lea & Febiger, Philadelphia, 1993.

To calculate your energy expenditure for your primary activity locate it on an energy expenditure table, then refer to the column that comes closest to your body weight. Look across from your primary activity and down from your body weight and you will see the energy cost of that activity in calories per minute. Multiply the calories per minute by the number of minutes you exercise.

For example, if the 140-pound exerciser we referred to earlier goes for a cross-training run at a pace of 11:30 per mile (5.2 miles per hour), you can see on the Table that the runner is expending about 8.8 calories per minute. This converts to 176 calories for a 20-minute run.

If your cross-training option is swimming, you can see the energy expenditure differs by stroke. Our exerciser weighs in at 140 pounds and is doing the crawl stroke slowly. He or she will be expending approximately 8.3 calories per minute. To make this swim workout equal to the run workout in terms of energy expenditure the swim would have to last for 21 minutes (176 calories ÷ 8.3 cal/min = 21.2 minutes).

Let's look at Katie (140 pounds) doing aerobic dance at high intensity and cross training with cycling at about 9.4 miles per hour. Katie is expending approximately 8.7 calories per minute during her 30-minute aerobic dance workouts, for a total of 261 calories. When she cycles she is expending about 6.7 calories per minute so she needs to ride for 39 minutes to match the calories expended during her dance class.

You can perform any of these simple comparisons and calculations for your cross-training activities. Record your results in your training log (discussed in chapter 13). Knowing how your workouts compare will give you additional confidence as you add new activities to your cross-training program.

Computer Programs for Cross Training

Recording the details of your workouts on a computer program can be fun and useful. It's fun because you get a feeling of achievement as you type in the numbers that represent your effort. It's useful because after you print it out it is easier to compare one workout to another.

The Athlete's Diary (Stevens Creek Software, 21346 Rumford Drive, Cupertino, CA 95014) uses a spreadsheet so you can track your activity in eight different sports. You can look at mileage per month, average miles per week, and several other combinations of training information.

The Athlete's Log (B & B Software, Inc., P.O. Box 10212, Eugene, OR 97440) is excellent if your sports include swimming, biking, or running. The Athlete's Log has an excellent calendar format. It also allows you to describe courses that you use regularly and the program will automatically fill in the mileage.

Fitness Tracker (Lunde Engineering, Inc., 5154 North 90th Street, Omaha, NE 68134) is a training-log database. It's easy to install, easy to use, and produces attractive, easy to read graphs. The program can be used for any activity, which makes it especially valuable for cross-training athletes.

Staying Healthy

A s discussed earlier, cross training cuts down on trauma to the body caused by excessive training and therefore reduces the possibility and frequency of overuse injuries. Cross training has also been identified by Dr. Mary O'Toole of the Department of Orthopedic Surgery at the University of Tennessee as one of five strategies for treating injured endurance athletes. The strategies are: 1) appropriate medical care; 2) athlete education; 3) cross training; 4) specific exercises; 5) programmed return to activity.

This chapter will not, however, focus on details of self-treatment. There are excellent books available with such information. One is *Sports Fitness and Training* by Richard Mangi, Peter Jokl, and O. William Dayton (Pantheon Books, 1987).

What you will learn here is a ten-point approach to

staying healthy. In this context healthy refers to absence of injury, and injury is defined as any condition that causes you to exercise less than you do normally.

Ten Points for Staying Healthy

1. Listen to your body.

When you do a workout, whatever your activity or sport, there are sensations you feel. For example, to perform any aerobic activity at target heart rate zone intensity you will first breathe more deeply (a greater volume of oxygen goes into your body), then you will breathe more often (another way to get more oxygen to the lungs). While these two responses are occurring, your heart will gradually beat faster, taking the oxygen-rich blood from the lungs and pumping it to the working muscles.

As the body makes these adjustments, anyone, even a veteran exercise, can experience a few moments early in an aerobic workout during which he or she feels "out of breath." This feeling is a normal physiological response. You may interpret the breathlessness as a scary, somewhat painful symptom and think, This exercise stuff is just not for me. But beginning exercisers who stay with aerobic workouts of appropriate intensity soon discover that the temporary feeling of breathlessness is not dangerous at all. It passes quickly as the body goes into steady state—the oxygen delivered equals the oxygen needed.

This information, that the feeling of breathlessness is OK, becomes part of your physiological memory bank. As you do more workouts this bank takes in more information. Cross training broadens the bank because you experience new movements and sensations as you do new activities. You become finely attuned to what you can do safely.

When you are in the early stages of building your physiological memory bank you will learn some of the lessons the hard way, which is to say, you will have injuries. But if you are in touch with what feels acceptable and what feels unusual, you may be able to keep the injury to a minimum. It's the athlete who *ignores* the unusual pain again and again who ends up with a chronic injury followed by rehabilitation.

Listen for acute (sharp) pain. Whether in a muscle, joint, tendon or ligament, acute pain must be taken seriously. Either slow down or stop. If the pain goes away completely within 24 to 48 hours you can try doing your next workout, but begin slowly. If the pain returns as you move you should consider getting an opinion from a medical professional familiar with your activity or sport.

As you learn to listen to your body you will learn how to ease into a new activity. You will be able to tell when you are ready to go hard. You will know when it's time to slow down. Listening to your body will teach you how to distinguish between minor aches and pains and more serious signs of tissue damage. You will be able to tell when you need to rest—whether for a day or a week or a month. Of course, if you need a month off from one activity you may well be cross training with another during that time.

Resting as needed is just as important as any principle of exercise. Being well rested before you begin a workout assures that you will be able to enjoy the workout. The delicate aspect of recommending rest pertains to beginning exercisers who are trying to integrate exercise into their lives and finding they are unintentionally skipping workouts. Letting your workout fall to a low priority should not be mistaken for taking a day off to rest. If you are striving to exercise consistently, and you're not tired, then get busy and do your workout as planned. If you wake up feeling sluggish and there's no change by the time you are supposed to exercise—that's different. In this case it's all right to take a day off. Missing any one workout for a legitimate reason is not something to fret about. Think of yourself as an athlete planning on a long, healthy career.

2. Think long term.

Think long term. A professional sports general manager says he is thinking long term when he announces "I have a five-year plan that will turn this team around." The young executive says "In ten years I will be a vice-president." How do you feel about exercise as a long-term proposition?

You should be thinking long term whether you are twenty or seventy. How old are you now? How long would you like to live? Average age expectancy keeps going up for men and women. Let's suppose you are going to have a forty-year cross-training career. The first immediate benefit that comes from thinking long term is the realization that you can take a day off when you need to rest—and not feel guilty about it.

With a long-term view, if you ever do get hurt, knowing that you will be exercising for many years will help you cope with your injury. It is helpful if you think of recovery time in terms of a few weeks versus a forty-year exercise career. You will probably be more willing to wait for the doctor's OK to exercise again rather than trying to rush back to your workouts before your body is ready.

Thinking long term is also an excellent approach to take when you are contemplating your own commitment to exercise.

3. Develop sound technique.

"We think injuries stem from improper mechanics," says Dr. Louis Bigliani of the Columbia-Presbyterian Center for Sports Medicine in New York City. "When you're doing something over and over again minor things [incorrect technique] can lead to injuries."

Tennis elbow, or tendinitis of the elbow, provides an example of the value of sound technique. One way a player gets tennis elbow is hitting a backhand with a floppy wrist. In a survey of more than a thousand people who had recovered from tennis elbow, the players were asked what finally had cured them. The leading answer, by far? Tennis lessons.

Lessons have been recommended for many of the activities and sports discussed in this book. When you learn how to do a given movement properly you establish sound biomechanics.

Another reason to concentrate on biomechanics is that poor form often hinders improvement.

How Can You Develop Sound Technique?

- Watch experts and see if they are doing something you should copy.
- Read about the finer points of your skill and apply what you learn to your practice sessions.
- Have a friend videotape you and study the tape. Seeing yourself move may help you make needed adjustments.
- Buy an instructional videotape.
- Be a student of your game. You'll get it right—and prevent injury—if you work on better technique.

4. Use quality equipment.

You'd be surprised how many well-intentioned exercisers get off on the wrong foot by wearing the wrong exercise shoes. The Reebok Company has made a legitimate contribution to the physical well-being of millions of active Americans by introducing cross-training footwear.

In my fifteen years as an exercise physiologist I have advised many new members to purchase footwear appropriate to their activities. Not long ago if you wanted to jog and play tennis you needed two different pairs of exercise shoes. Many people hurt themselves because they were unwilling to put up the money for the second pair of shoes (or they didn't realize that the type of shoe truly affects the safety of your activity).

Tell the salesperson your needs so you can purchase the cross-training shoe designed for your exercise combinations.

Cyclists should wear a helmet to protect themselves against a situation that cannot be anticipated. We call these situations accidents—and they can happen to anyone. It is not a negative reflection on your cycling skills, judgment, or bravery to put on a helmet when you go out for a ride. It is a mark of good common sense.

Be smart. Whatever your sport, be sure your equipment fits, know how to use your equipment correctly, and always think, Safety first.

5. Respect your training threshold.

In this situation training threshold means: How much exercise can you do safely? Every athlete has a limit for his or her activity. When you do more than your limit, when you go beyond your training threshold, injuries start to happen.

If you are one of the many active Americans who enjoys exercise in moderate doses you may not ever have to deal with this type of training threshold—and as a reward for your good judgment you'll have a healthier exercise career.

If you are in another, sizable group of exercisers, those who can't resist the thought process that says more is better and lots more is even better, you may end up discovering your training threshold—and you will almost definitely pay the price of an injury. (Exercisers who follow Point 1—Listen to your body—may be able to cut back on their activity *just before* the onset of injury.)

Here's a typical scenario. You love your activity or sport. You do it every chance you get. You are doing a lot of workouts and one day you feel some pain. You don't pay any attention to the pain; you are hoping it will go away by itself. You keep exercising and the pain is getting worse. You continue to ignore it. Finally the pain is so strong that you have to stop. You go for a diagnosis, you get treatment, you begin some type of rehabilitation. Now, here's the question. What did you learn from this experience? If you are bright, you learn to recognize when to *cut back* on your workouts so that you don't get hurt. If you have a training diary (Point 10) it will be easier for you to go back and trace your workouts so you can see when you hit your training threshold.

Let's look at two general examples of training thresholds. Many sports medicine physicians have said that for recreational runners twenty miles per week seems to be a training threshold. When these runners keep their weekly mileage under twenty miles per week they stay healthy. If you are or want to be a distance runner there is a good chance that you will end up discovering what your training threshold is. If you do learn it, respect it.

Starting pitchers in major league baseball usually throw in a game only once every four or five days.

Repeatedly throwing a baseball at 80 to 100 miles per hour damages the arm, elbow, and shoulder, and therefore the pitcher needs a few days off to rest. Some pitchers can perform and stay healthy with three days rest; others need four days rest. The manager, the pitching coach, and the pitcher all need to know the training threshold as it applies to days off between starts.

Managers assign a pitcher taking a rest day to chart and count the number of pitches his teammate is throwing. Some pitchers can throw more pitches than others without getting hurt. Again, the training threshold for each pitcher is important.

Be aware of how much you are doing in your activity. Learn when to end a workout and when to take a day off.

6. Warm up and cool down Properly

There are two aspects to a proper warm-up: increasing blood flow and stimulating neuromuscular pathways. Many physiologists recommend a proper warm-up for purposes of injury prevention. However, a 1990 study at the University of California-San Diego indicated that the pain and swelling that occasionally afflicts joggers, cyclists, and other athletes resulted, in most cases, from torn muscle fibers. This tearing did not result from a lack of oxygen to the muscle, the researchers say, therefore warming up will not prevent it. Since there has not been enough research done on this subject to make a definitive statement for or against the traditional warm-up, I have chosen to include it as a means of preventing injury (if not soreness).

For many activities you can accomplish both aspects of the warm-up simultaneously. The swimmer who does the first few laps slowly is warming up properly. Some boxers prefer to divide their warm-up into two parts. First they jump rope to increase blood circulation, then they hit the speed bag and the heavy bag to stimulate the specific neuromuscular pathways involved in the skill of boxing.

Your cooldown is important too. During the cooldown you should be doing movements that permit your blood to redistribute throughout your body. If you were doing some type of lower body activity such as vigorous ice skating and you stopped suddenly, your blood would pool in your lower extremities. Skate for a few minutes slowly at the end of your workout. After your skates are off walk for a few minutes. Gently stretch the muscles that were doing most of the work.

Whatever your activity, cool down properly when you are done.

7. Consider Mother Nature.

Try not to exercise when it's very hot outside, but if you do take these precautions:

- Wear loose, light-colored clothing, including a hat.
- Drink plenty of fluids before you work out, and replenish water lost through perspiration by taking drinks every fifteen to thirty minutes throughout your workout.
- Adjust your intensity and take it easy if the heat is draining your energy level.
- Shorten your workout if you feel tired or overheated.
- Replace magnesium, potassium, and the other minerals lost through sweating by increasing your intake of bananas, watermelon, cantaloupe, carrots, tomatoes, or commercially produced electrolyte drinks.
- Depending on your activity, it may be appropriate to use a sun protection product on your skin.
- If you feel dizzy or uncomfortable in any way that strikes you as unusual, get out of the sun right away. If you don't feel better, seek medical attention.

If you are going to exercise in the cold:

- Wear layers to trap the heat produced by your body. The inner layer should be absorbent (a cotton tee-shirt is good). The next layer should be a light material such as polypropylene, and then put on a sweatshirt. The outermost layer should be a waterproof windbreaker.
- One layer of clothing may be enough for your legs, but if you feel you need a second layer don't hesitate. You will enjoy your run more if you are warm; you won't enjoy it if you feel chilled.
- Cover your head! Use vaseline on your face, wear a ski mask, a woolen hat, or a headband. Wear gloves, mittens, or even socks on your hands.
- Watch your step if there is snow or ice on the ground.

Shorten your stride or otherwise adjust your pace so you don't fall.

8. Eat the right food at the right time.

You can diminish the quality of a given workout if you don't pay attention to what and when you are eating.

Many morning exercisers find they need only a light breakfast—juice and a small bowl of cereal, for example—before an early workout. Other exercisers have a late dinner, exercise enjoyably the next morning, and have breakfast after the workout.

You should not have a large, heavy meal just before a workout. When there is a lot of food in your stomach blood is shunted to the stomach to aid in the digestive process. This means there is less blood available to help the muscles do their work. You are likely to feel sluggish as you try to work out.

Another scenario to avoid is going all day without eating and then trying to do your workout. You run the risk of getting dizzy. Have a light meal and wait an hour, then you will be able to have a good workout.

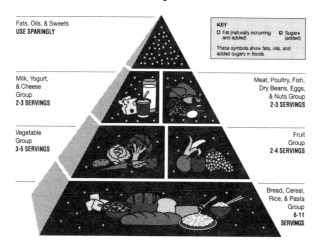

Food Guide Pyramid
A Guide to Daily Food Choices

(Reprinted by permission. U.S. Department of Agriculture, Human Nutrition Information Service, August 1992.)

9. Keep a diary.

When cross training keeping a diary is a great idea. You will have fun recording your different activities. You will comment on how different combinations feel and, over a period of time, you will put together various workout mixes.

The advantage of your diary from a "stay healthy" perspective is this: If you do feel something is not right with your body you can look at your notes and may be able to figure out what is causing the discomfort. Every physician is trained to do this before treating you. The doctor asks questions to learn what has happened before. (*Note:* For any sharp, serious, or persistent pain seek professional medical care immediately.)

However, as you learn to listen to your body you may be able to solve certain minor problems on your own.

Diaries vary in the information recorded. Look at the categories listed below and decide for yourself which categories interest you enough that you will be willing to record workout details faithfully.

Day/date/time of day:

Aerobic activity or activities:

Distance or results:

Time spent on each section of the workout:

Stretching routine:

Strength-training routine:

Body weight:

Morning resting heart rate:

Feeling:

General comments:

10. For medical advice, talk to a sports medicine expert.

Sports medicine is not part of the standard medical school curriculum. When it comes to treating exercise-related injuries, many well-meaning doctors who are not athletes and who have not studied sports medicine have little choice but to say you should stop exercising. What you should have is a doctor who will take the trouble to learn how you were injured and what to do to prevent the injury from recurring.

Dr. James G. Garrick, an orthopedist at the Center for Sports Medicine at St. Francis Hospital in San Francisco also recommends that exercisers see an expert. As he puts it, "Anyone can give you antiinflammatory drugs and tell you to rest. You should demand more than that."

14

Crossroads

I n his poem "The Road Not Taken" Robert Frost discusses the life implications stemming from the decision to choose one road instead of another. As you head down your own boulevard of life you intersect with many roads—one of which is the road that includes exercise. The beauty of this road is that you can be on it without changing course. You simply *add* it to your route. In fact, there is an excellent chance that if you do become a regular exerciser, your life journey will be much better for doing so.

For Those Who Have Never Exercised

People who are already in the habit of doing something are going to justify their actions by defending their behavior as logical, intelligent, and admirable. If you have been inactive to date, you may feel that if you announce you are going to begin exercising now, you were in error somehow *before*. Perhaps it's unpleasant to experience such an acknowledgement. But you can deal with this feeling.

Have you ever thought about why you didn't get into an exercise routine when you were a young adult? Could it be, when you were in your teens and early twenties, that you were moving all the time without ever having to schedule a workout for yourself? You had activities such as dancing, school gym class, cheerleading, and teams. You went away with friends to participate in other activities such as hiking, camping, white-water rafting, snow skiing, and horseback riding. Or you went to the beach to body surf, run in the waves, and play Frisbee. You had lots of time for recreation and sleeping late (you were easily able to get the rest needed to recover between activities). There was no reason for you to worry about your weight, physical fitness, or health.

What happened?

You finished your education, whether high school or college, you left home, and you took on real obligations such as a full-time job, parenting, or both. Perhaps you decided to continue your education while working. The schoolwork cut sharply into your personal time. Perhaps now you have to care for an older relative, too. Maybe you are involved with your child's school as a member of the P.T.A., or you are a volunteer speaker, or you chaperone class trips. You could be donating time to your professional organization by serving as an officer. The list of ways your day can be spent once you are past your mid-twenties can go on and on.

What is the point of mentioning all these important endeavors? By tracing the path you took away from a naturally active lifestyle you can see how you drifted away from exercise.

Did you ever make a rational and conscious decision, saying, "I do not like or need exercise—period"? If you never said that, then maybe you should ask yourself now, whether you are 30 or 80, did you enjoy being more active and more fit? If the answer is yes there is great news for you. You can be active and fit again. And along the way you may well *feel* younger, too.

Assuming you do think you would benefit from regular exercise, where will it fit into your weekly schedule? You probably like your weekly schedule as it is. To add regular exercise you will need to plan. You will need to apply the same intelligence you have used to succeed in school and at work and in other areas of your life to your workouts.

There is more to exercising as an adult than saying, "I really should be working out." There is more to it than paying for a health club membership or a class. But it's my impression that some well-intentioned people feel better about not exercising if they are at least paying for exercise. If you have been one of these people, please remember, you gotta be in it to win it, and you have to *do* your workouts to get the benefits.

Planning for Exercise

The questions that follow anticipate numerous possible scenarios. Skip the questions that don't apply to your situation. It's an excellent idea to sketch out your answers. Writing solutions can be helpful in crystallizing an action.

Planning cannot be amorphous. Think your answers through. Sit down and discuss the plan with your partner. You increase your chances of exercising consistently by doing some problem solving before you begin.

1. **Are you going to exercise for your own benefit, or for someone else's benefit?**
   It's fine if you are reading this book because it was given to you as a gift and the gesture has prompted you to start exercising. But in the end you are more likely to stay with your workouts if you are doing them for *you*. Others may take joy in the fact that you are taking care of yourself, and that's wonderful. You must take joy in your workouts, too.

2. **Should you have a medical examination before you begin exercising?**
   Here's what the American College of Sports Medicine says: Apparently healthy individuals are those who are

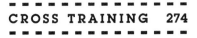

asymptomatic and apparently healthy with no more than one major coronary risk factor.

Major Coronary Risk Factors

1. Diagnosed hypertension or systolic blood pressure ≥ 160 or diastolic blood pressure ≥ 90 mmHg on at least two separate occasions, or on hypertensive medication
2. Serum cholesterol ≥ 6.20 millimoles/Liter (≥ 240 milligrams/deciliter)
3. Cigarette smoking
4. Diabetes mellitus
5. Family history of coronary or other atherosclerotic disease in patients or siblings prior to age 55

If you are in the "apparently healthy" category you can begin moderate exercise (target heart rate roughly 70 to 85 percent of maximum predicted heart rate—the formula is explained in chapter 3) without the need for exercise testing or a medical examination as long as the exercise program begins and proceeds gradually and as long as you are alert to the development of unusual signs or symptoms.

If you have had any symptoms or signs that suggest you should be examined by a physician before embarking on your exercise program, be smart and get the medical go-ahead first.

1. What type of exercise would you like to do?

Write down all your choices. Later you will sift through them to determine what's most practical and what will have to wait. Chapters 8 and 11 are replete with suggestions for sweating.

Exercise Choices

- - - - - - - - - - -

1. _____
2. _____
3. _____
4. _____
5. _____

6. _____
7. _____
8. _____
9. _____
10. _____

What can you afford?

Make some calls if you need information. Remember, any money put toward your exercise is money well spent. You are always wise to invest in your own health.

1. Will you need lessons to get started?

2. Will you need equipment?

3. Will you be taking out a membership at a club?

4. Will you pay dues to join an exercise organization so you can receive event notices—race applications, for example—and other news about your activity or sport?

5. Will you pay for classes?

6. Will you pay for court time?

7. Can you afford a personal trainer?

8. Will you be giving up income to begin exercising? This can be a tough choice. You must be able to meet expenses.

9. Could you gain income by exercising? Could you save on transportation expenses such as gas or fares by jogging, cycling, or in-line skating to work?

10. Can you afford a piece of home exercise equipment?

11. Will you have child-care expenses? Adults and friends can take turns with child care. Look for a club or Y that has a class for Junior while Mom or Dad works out.

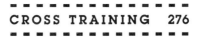

12. Where will you exercise?

    The more *yes* answers the better, because you give yourself more options.

    In your neighborhood?

    At an exercise facility at or near work?

    At a health club near home?

    Will you exercise when you travel for business?

    Will you exercise when you travel for pleasure?

13. What time of day will you exercise?

    "Whenever I have time" is too vague. You can change your workout time when necessary, but first you must select a specific time and block that time off for yourself.

    Before work?

    At lunch time?

    After work?

    If you are off from work, what time will you exercise?

    In some cities you can find health clubs that are open twenty-four hours a day.

Of course, even if you come up with feasible, terrific answers to all these exercise readiness questions, you are still up against one of the toughest challenges you will ever face: Behavior Change.

There are people who have had their larynx removed as a result of cigarette smoking and get caught by nurses in the hospital room doing what—you guessed it—smoking smuggled cigarettes through the stoma (the hole in their neck through which they have to breathe after the operation). Yet, as difficult as it can be to change any habit, people do change behavior all the time. Millions have stopped smoking in the past ten years. In counseling people trying to stop smoking I discovered a few things.

Many people do not succeed in stopping the first time they try. This is an important realization. If you try to add exercise to your weekly schedule and things don't work out, think about what prevented you from getting into a steady routine. When you are ready to make the necessary adjustments, do so and try again.

When you try to change a behavior you may find that you learn something about yourself. Be introspective.

Think about what makes you tick. What do you respond to? What turns you off? For your workouts, what was it that interfered with consistency? Was it your choice of exercise? Was it a logistics problem? Think the situation through and try again. You can do it and it will be worth it.

Dissociation

The physiological and psychological benefits of exercise are impressive, and there are exercisers who keep themselves going by intellectualizing the process. Some of my students and friends have explained to me that they know exercise is good for them and they are happy with the results of their workouts, but they just can't seem to find the workout itself as fun. A technique that can help if you have not yet come to revel in your routine in dissociation.

Dissociation is based on the idea that one can attend to only a limited number of stimuli at any given moment. One often-used example of dissociation is music. Try wearing headphones so you can listen to your favorite station or cassette tape while you do your workout. If you can set yourself up to exercise at home you can use a regular radio or the TV to provide dissociation.

Can you find an exercise partner? The conversation you have with a partner provides dissociation. Part of the popularity of personal trainers is the way they take your mind off the muscular effort. If you are fortunate enough to be able to afford a personal trainer such support will keep you going.

If you are riding a stationary bike or exercising on a step machine, set a low intensity and you may be able to read while you exercise.

Forty-two-year-old Rich Girgenti plans his day while running on the treadmill. You may like to think through areas of your work or home life so that your aerobic exercise time will pass easily.

If you do use headphones when running outside keep the music at a volume that allows you to hear what's going on around you. For example, if you are crossing a street and a car honks at you, you need to be able to hear it.

Dissociation may not be necessary at all if you come to

relish the ritual of rolling through your favorite exercise routine. It's to your great advantage if you are able to see your beading perspiration as the liquid of life and take pleasure in the *process* of the workout. Whether you shift your focus away from your muscles or on to each contraction, you will devise a mindset that will take you through each workout.

Goal Setting

Goal setting is extremely powerful because so much of human achievement is a self-fulfilling prophecy. Can you see yourself as slim and trim? Can you see yourself walking or running or cycling or climbing or stepping or skating? Why not? You can do it. You don't need to be as fast as Carl Lewis. You don't need to have the all-around athletic ability of Olympic champion heptathlete Jackie Joyner-Kersey. Be your own athlete. As the army slogan says "Be all that you can be."

New York City psychologist Dr. Gerard Shaw specializes in helping athletes achieve their goals. Here are his guidelines for successful goal setting, supplemented by my insights on their relevance to cross training:

1. Make your goals challenging but realistic.

Set goals that are not easy but are attainable. If you are going to cross train by adding a new sport that involves head-to-head competition, your first challenge might be to perform respectably at the beginner's level. You will define this level for yourself.

If you are adding in-line skating to your weekly workouts, for example, you can set a goal of skating for twenty minutes without falling down.

2. Be specific about your goals.

Here's a good specific goal: On Saturday I will go down to the health club and find out what they have to offer, what the hours are, and the membership costs. Or: "I want to add strength training to my routine and I want to do it at home. I will go to the sporting goods store and buy a set of barbells and dumbbells when they have the next sale."

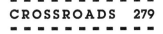

3. Set measurable goals.

"I will do three regular workouts this week and one with just stretching" is a measurable goal.

4. Set your own goals.

As discussed earlier, you have a far better chance to succeed when you work toward accomplishing your own objectives. If you are the first on your block to understand cross training you may hear some skepticism. It's not hard to imagine golfing partners advising you, "Geez, Joe, you can't run the ball into the hole" or "Mary, if you have time for anything you should spend it practicing putting in the living room." Your friends may not be able to fathom that your goal in cross training with golf is not to lower your score but to enjoy another type of exercise and be healthier. Regardless of anyone else's support, or lack thereof, set your own goals, stay with them, be pleased when you achieve them.

5. Work within a time frame.

Give yourself a target date to work toward. "I would like to complete the Peoria 5K [3.1 miles] Walk/Run Fund Raiser on June 1." "I will add one lap to my swim workout each Monday for the next eight weeks."

6. Be flexible.

When you can't get to the squash court because you had to finish a report for the boss you try to go the next day. And if you don't have a reservation for the court the next day you can cross train with another activity.

7. Write down your goals.

Written goals are more concrete, and many people make a better commitment to a new endeavor when they put it in writing.

There is also a benefit in record keeping. When you look back at your notes from time to time you will find it gratifying to see how much you have done. If you are in need of encouragement you just might say to yourself, "I did it before [got in to good shape], I can do it again."

8. Prioritize.

You may have multiple goals. You may want to start aerobic dance class, improve muscle tone, fit into a size 10, and be able to play three sets of tennis comfortably. Think through what you need to do first to begin working toward these goals.

Alternate Behavior

You can integrate greater physical activity into your day even if you are not yet ready for full-fledged cross-training workouts. Goal setting fits in well here as you look for opportunities to be more active. Once you decide on the new behavior you set your goal to do it.

For example, if you wish to walk sixty minutes per week and you drive to work each day, perhaps you could park your car about a half a mile away from work. You walk ten minutes on the way to your job and you walk ten minutes back at the end of the day. You will expend about 100 to 125 calories per day beyond your typical metabolic output, and you'll be healthier. You could begin with three days per week and, if you are enjoying your walks and the weather is good, go to four or five. Maybe you have co-workers who would like to park near you so you could walk to work together.

Have you thought about taking the stairs whenever possible instead of the elevator? Your goal could be to walk one flight of stairs the first week and add one flight every two weeks until you get to five. Eric Drucker, special assistant to the director of personnel at John Jay College, lost fifteen pounds and lowered his cholesterol by eighty points by taking the stairs at every opportunity throughout his work-day.

When you go to the beach you should do more than sunbathe. Go for a walk or a jog along the water's edge.

Bringing the Family
Into the Cross Training World

Another terrific goal is to get the family involved. Everyone in your family will be happier and healthier if they enjoy exercise. There are only a few values you can instill in your

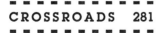

children more important than the desire to take care of one's well being. Here is a story illustrating one idea for a family outing which included exercise.

The Tuxedo 10K

For years my wife Litna and I would go apple picking each fall at the Mascar Orchards in Muncy, New York. While I am always happy to be with Litna, apple picking was not one of my own family childhood activities and I viewed the excursion as one of those things husbands must do from time to time (Litna came to all my games when I was coaching so fair is fair).

Once we added Danny, Katie and Rebecca to our family these outings took on a new spirit and I had come to see the annual apple picking as great fun for the kids.

Then in 1990, we were only twenty minutes from the orchards while driving along Route 17A when I saw a big sign which gave me an idea: "Tuxedo 10K". Later that week I called the Recreation Office of the town of Tuxedo and asked to be put on the mailing list for the 1991 race. When the application came in August I noticed right away that besides the 6.2 mile race, there was a ½ mile fun run for children and parents. I suggested to Litna we do the race and the fun run first and then continue to the orchards for the apple picking. Alas, race day was rained out.

We tried to make the Tuxedo 10K event again in 1992. By then we were doing group activities with our friends Nelson and Debbie Serrano, who had been cross training all summer and had done a couple of 5Ks (3.1 miles) together. They were excited about the challenge of the longer distance. Neighbor Mary Fava and her five-year-old Danny would join Litna, our Danny, and Katie for the Fun Run. Mary's husband, Pat, and I were on baby patrol.

We met at the corner of our block at 8:00 A.M. sharp on 10K/Fun Run/apple-picking day and, even with a little car trouble, made it to the race start in plenty of time. Do you know what? Everyone thoroughly enjoyed the race and Fun Run. The children got ribbons, the parents got great workouts, and Litna and Mary vowed to train enough to do the whole 6.2 miles with Debbie in 1993.

What events and excursions would your family enjoy? There is planning involved, whether the outing includes physical activity or not. If you make up your mind you want the family to be active you will find a way to make it happen.

Certain activities seem to fit with families more easily than others and they are listed below, but don't limit yourself to these ideas. Use your own imagination and get everyone involved.

Family Activity Ideas

- Family Bowling Outing

    Bowling has its strikes and splits, but it's better than the couch. Try to go easy on the french fries between spares. Chapter Six has a few cross training for bowling ideas.
- Family Golf Outing
- Family Goes Outdoors Outing

    Backpacking, camping, hiking, orienteering—See Chapter Six subsection, "Going Wild in the Wilderness" for suggestions.
- Family Playground Outing

    The kids play. At the same time if you have another family with you, one or more adults can walk or jog around the park while the other adult supervises.
- Family Racquet Sport Workout

    Lessons for Junior while Mom and Dad relive The Challenge of the Sexes? Mixed doubles? See what you can come up with which gives everybody a shot.
- Family Goes Rowing Outing

    One rule: When switching oarsmen, no one is allowed to fall out of the boat.
- Family Sailing Outing

    And if you own your sailboat, the whole family can get a good workout by doing the maintenance.
- Family Reunion Soccer Match

    You will need more family members for this one. Put down a few sweatshirts, or rubber cones, and in five minutes you will have your field boundaries. Let the children take the midfield positions so they can

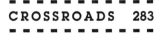

scamper up and down the field. Less-conditioned adults can substitute in for one another as needed.
- Family Swim Workout
    A big winner.
- Family Touch Football Game
    Tell the dads to cool their competitive juices and this will be an exciting event. Blocking not allowed.
- Family Volleyball Game
    Let the younger children catch and throw the ball.
- Family Walk, Jog, Run Workout
    Go around the block together. Or for a more organized workout, take the family to the local track. We bring the kids' bikes and they can do laps on a quarter mile track. Our seven-year-old, Danny, was very proud to announce he rode three miles during a track outing last summer.

Crossroads

In the end, for most adults and families, whether cross training is included as a significant part of their lives is determined by the will power of the individuals involved. This is not to say you have no willpower if you have been inactive. It means that if you make up your mind that you want to discover, enjoy, and reap the many benefits of cross training, you surely will.

As I did the research for this book I was struck by a recurring theme. All the authors whose books I read professed great love for their sports and they each made at least one argument why their sport was the very best. Which will be the best sport or activity for you? As you know by now, I am suggesting that in the long run you will be best off, and happiest, with a combination of activities. There are many wonderful sports and activities from which to choose. Find the combinations which reward you the most.

Cross Training presents a philosophical and practical approach to exercise:

Be balanced.
Think long term.
Enjoy your workouts.

Appendix

Appendix A
Potential Physical Fitness Benefits Provided by Activities and Sports

| Activity/Sport | Aerobic Capacity | Strength | | Flexibility | | Total |
		Upper Body	Lower Body	Upper Body	Lower Body	
aerobic dance	4	2	4*	3	4	17
backpacking	3	3	3	1	3	13
badminton	3	2	3	4	3	15
ballet (men)	3	4**	4	4	4	19
ballet (women)	3	2	4	4	4	17
baseball	2***	4	3	3	3	15
basketball	4	3	4	3	3	17
bowling	1	2	1	3	2	9
boxing	4	4	4	4	3	19
canoeing	4	4	1	4	1	14

*4 for high impact, 3 for low impact
**4 for men because they do lifts
***aerobic benefits vary according to position and from game to game

Rating Scale

4 = excellent 3 = good 2 = fair 1 = minimal

Activity/Sport	Aerobic Capacity	Strength Upper Body	Strength Lower Body	Flexibility Upper Body	Flexibility Lower Body	Total
climbing machine	4	4	4	3	3	18
cross-country skiing	4	4	4	4	4	20
cross-country ski machine	4	3	3	3	3	16
cycling	4	3	4	3	3	17
cycling (stationary bike)	4	1	4	2	2	13
folk dance	3	2	3	2	2	12
golf	2	3	2	4	2	13
handball	4	2	3	4	3	16
in-line skating	4	2	4	2	3	15
judo	2	4	4	4	4	18
jumping rope	4	3	4	3	2	16
karate	2	3	4	4	4	17
orienteering	4*	2	4	2	2	14
paddleball	4	2	3	4	3	16
racquetball	4	2	3	4	3	16

* when performed competitively

Rating Scale

4 = excellent   3 = good   2 = fair   1 = minimal

Activity/Sport	Aerobic Capacity	Strength		Flexibility		Total
		Upper Body	Lower Body	Upper Body	Lower Body	
rowing	4	4	4	4	3	19
rowing machine	4	4	4	3	2	17
running	4	2	4	2	2	14
slide boarding	4	2	3	2	3	14
snowboarding	3	1	3	1	2	10
squash	4	2	3	4	3	16
step class	4	2	4	3	4	17
step machine	4	1	4	1	2	12
swimming	4	4	3	4	3	18
tennis (singles)	4	3	4	4	4	19
tennis (doubles)	3	3	3	4	3	16
triathlon	4	4	4	4	3	19
walking	3	1	2	1	2	9
water exercise	3	3	2	2	3	13
water running	4	2	3	2	3	14

Rating Scale

4 excellent   3 = good   2 = fair   1 = minimal

Appendix B
Activities & Sports Ranked
by Potential Physical Fitness Benefits

Minimum score = 5   Maximum score = 20

Activity/Sport	Physical Fitness Benefits Index
cross-country skiing	20
ballet (for men)	19
boxing	19
rowing	19
tennis (singles)	19
triathlon	19
judo	18
swimming	18
climbing machine	18
aerobic dance (high impact)	17
ballet (women)	17
basketball	17
cycling	17
karate	17
rowing machine	17
step class	17
aerobic dance (low impact)	16
cross-country ski machine	16
handball	16
jump rope	16
paddleball	16
racquetball	16
squash	16
tennis (doubles)	16
badminton	15
baseball	15
in-line skating	15
canoeing	14
running	14

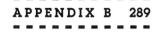

Activity/Sport	Physical Fitness Benefits Index
orienteering	14
slide boarding	14
water running	14
backpacking	13
golf	13
water exercise	13
cycling (stationary bike)	13
folk dance	12
step machine	12
snowboarding	10
walking	9
bowling	9

Appendix C
Exercise Organizations

Amateur Athletic Union
3400 West 86th Street
Indianapolis, IN 46268

American College of Sports Medicine
P.O. Box 1440
Indianapolis, IN 46206

American Hiking Society
1015 31st Street, N.W.
Washington, D.C. 20007

American National Red Cross
17th and D Streets, N.W.
Washington, D.C. 20006

American Running and Fitness Association
20001 S Street, N.W., Suite 540
Washington, D.C. 20009

Bicycle Federation of America
1818 R Street, N.W.
Washington, D.C. 20009

Cooper Institute for Aerobic Research
12330 Preston Road
Dallas, TX 75230

International In-Line Skating Association
3033 Excelsior Blvd., Suite 300
Minneapolis, MN 55416

Masters Sports
P.O. Box 3000
Denville, NJ 07834–3000

National Strength Conditioning Association
P.O. Box 81410
Lincoln, NE 68501

New York Road Runners Club
9 East 89th Street
New York, NY 10128

Powerlifting USA
P.O. Box 467
Camarillo, CA 93011

President's Council on Physical Fitness and Sports
Department of Health and Human Services
450 5th Street, N.W.
Washington, D.C. 20001

Prevention Walking Club
Rodale Press
Box 6099
Emmaus, PA 18099

Rockport Walking Institute
P.O. Box 480
Marlboro, MA 01752

Tri-Fed USA
National Office
P.O. Box 15820
Colorado Springs, CO 80935–5828

U.S. Cycling Federation
1750 East Boulder Street
Colorado Springs, CO 80909

U.S. Masters Swimming
5 Piggott Lane
Avon, CT 06001

U.S. Swimming, Inc.
1750 E. Boulder Street
Colorado Springs, CO 80909

U.S. Weightlifting Federation
U.S. Olympic Complex
1750 E. Boulder Street
Colorado Springs, CO 80909

Walking Association
Box 37228
Tucson, AZ 85740

Walkways Center
733 15th Street, N.W.
Washington, D.C. 20005

Selected References

American College of Sports Medicine: *Guidelines for Exercise Testing and Prescription*, 4th Edition. Philadelphia: Lea & Febiger, 1991.

Atkinson G and Bengtsson H: *Orienteering*. Brattleboro, VT: Stephen Greene Press, 1977.

Bartelski K: *Learn Downhill Skiing In A Weekend*. London: Dorling Kindersley Limited, 1992.

Bowers RW, Fox EL and Foss ML: *The Physiological Basis of Physical Education and Athletics*, Fourth Edition. Philadelphia: Saunders College Publishing, 1988.

Brady M: *Ski Cross Country*, New York: The Dial Press, 1982.

Brody J: Water Aerobics. *The New York Times*, April 4, 1991.

Brown B: *Stroke!*, Camden, Maine: International Marine Publishing Company, 1986.

Burfoot A: Stepping Up. *Runner's World*, December 1990.

Clarke M and Crisp C: *Understanding Ballet*. New York: Harmony Books, 1976.

Corbin C and Lindsey R: *Concepts of Physical Fitness*, 7th edition. Dubuque, Iowa, 1990.

DiGennaro J: *The New Physical Fitness: Exercise for Everybody*. Morton Publishing Company: Englewood, CO, 1983.

Downey J: *Winning Badminton Singles*. EP Publishing Limited: Wakefield, Great Britain, 1982.

Drotar D: *Hiking*. Stone Wall Press, Inc.: Washington, D.C., 1984.

Euser B: *Take 'em along: Sharing the Wilderness with your Children*. Evergreen, CO: Cordillera Press, 1987.

Feineman N: *Wheel Excitement*. New York: Hearst Books, 1991.

Fonda J: *Workout Book*. New York: Simon & Schuster, 1981.

Foster L: *Mountaineering Basics*. San Diego: Avant Books, 1982.

Fox R: *Basketball - The Complete Handbook of Individual Skills*. Englewood Cliffs, NJ: 1988.

Grant G: *Technical Manual and Dictionary of Classical Ballet*. New York: Dover Publications, 1967.

Gregory J: *Understanding BALLET*. London: Octopus Books, 1972.

Hagerman G: *Efficiency Racquet Sports*. New York: Bantam Books, 1987.

Harrison D: *Canoeing*. New York: Winner's Circle Books, 1988.

Jerome J: *Staying Supple, The Bountiful Pleasures of Stretching*. New York: Bantam Books, 1987.

Johnson J and Snead JC: *Golf Today*. St. Paul, MN: West Publishing Company, 1989.

Katch F and McArdle WD: *Nutrition, Weight Control and Exercise*. Philadelphia: Lea & Febiger, 1988.

Katz J: *Swimming For Total Fitness*. New York: Doubleday, 1981.

Katz J: *Swim 30 Laps In 30 Days*. New York: Perigee Books, 1991.

Klinger et al: *The Complete Encyclopedia of Aerobics*. Ithaca, NY: Mouvement Publications, 1986.

Kuntzleman C: *Rowing Machine Workouts*. Chicago: Contemporary Books, 1985.

LeMond G: *Complete Book of Bicycling*. New York: The Putnam Publishing Group, 1990.

Mara T: *First Step in Ballet*. Princeton: Princeton Book Company, 1987.

McDowell J: *Backpacking*. New York: Winner's Circle Books, 1989.

Mulvoy M: *Golf: Play Like A Pro*. New York: Winner's Circle Books, 1988.

Nieman D: *Fitness and Sports Medicine*. Palo Alto, CA: Bull Publishing Company, 1990.

Oates J: *On Boxing*. New York: Zebra Books, 1987.

Riley D: *Maximum Muscular Fitness, Strength Training Without Equipment*. West Point: Leisure Press, 1982.

Scott D: *Triathlon Training*. New York: Simon & Schuster, 1986.

Sheahan C: *Cross Country Skiing*. New York: Harper & Row, Publishers, 1984.

Sorenson J: *Aerobic Lifestyle Book*. New York: Poseidon Press, 1983.

Walker K: *Rock Climbing*. London: Dorling Kindersley Limited, 1991.

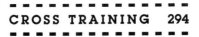

Wilmoth S: *Leading Aerobic Dance Exercise.* Champaign, IL: Human Kinetics, 1986.

Wiren G: *Golf: Building A Solid Game.* Englewood Cliffs, NJ: Prentice-Hall, Inc., 1987.

Index

Page numbers in *italics* refer to illustrative material: charts, drawings, photographs, and tables.

Balboa, Rocky, 114
Ballet
  exercise prescription for,
    235
  getting started in, 234–35
  positions in, precision of,
    232
  Potential Physical Fitness
    Benefits chart, for men,
    233; for women, 234
Baryshnikov, Mikhail, 225
Baseball
  benefits of cross training
    for, 99
  history of, 97–98
  jumping rope to improve
    throwing in, 101
  pitchers, training thresh-
    old of, 267
  physical fitness benefits
    of, 97–98
  Potential Physical Fitness
    Benefits chart for, 98
  prescription for cross
    training for, 99
  quickness and reflexes in,
    cross training to im-
    prove, 104–5
  skills in, cross training to
    improve, 97
  Sprint for the Cycle Work-
    out Table, 103–4
  sprint workout to improve
    speed in, 101–4
  strength training to im-
    prove hitting in, 100–
    101
  Strength Training Table
    for, 101
Basic Metabolic Rate
  (BMR), defined, 251

Basketball
  abdominal exercises for,
    110
  for baseball, to maintain
    quickness and reflexes
    in, 105
  cross training for, illus-
    trated, 107
  Cross training Program
    for, 106
  "Dream Team" in Olym-
    pics, 106–7
  history of, 106, 107
  Off-season Training Pro-
    gram for, 109
  pre-season cross training
    for, 113
  Potential Physical Fitness
    Benefits chart for, 108
  quickness in, cross train-
    ing for, 112–13
  speed in, cross training
    for, 110–12
  speed workout for, 110,
    111, 112
  strength in, cross training
    for, 108–10
Bell, Sam, 183
Bench, Johnny, 105
Bench Press Test, 81
Bench Press Test rating
  charts, for men, 82; for
  women, 83
Benoit-Samuelson, Joan,
  183
Bensimhon, Dan, 148
Bicycle Institute of America,
  211
Bicycles. See Cycling; Exercise bikes, indoor; Triathlon

Functional fitness, 25, 42–43, 45; 8–12
    Double Variable Routine recommended for, 50, and women, 45

Garrick, Dr. James G., 271
Gichin, Funakoshi, 122
Girgenti, Rich, 278
Golf
    aerobic activities for, 119–20
    flexibility, exercises for, 118
    Potential Physical Fitness Benefits of, 119
    strength, cross training for, 119
Golf Today (J. C. Snead and John Johnson), 118
Gratton, Mike, 9
Gravitron, 74–75, 143
Gray's Anatomy, 39
Guernsey, Rev. Jesse, 236

Handball, Potential Physical Fitness Benefits chart for, 127
Handy, Jam, 178
Hansen, Joy, 9
Harrison, Dave (Canoeing: Skills for the Serious Paddler), 240
Heart
    benefits to, with aerobic exercise, 11
    cardiac muscle of, 42

coronary risk factors, major, 275
defined, 251
and exercise heart rate, how to calculate, 15, 16
rate as measurement of workout intensity, 254
and stress test, 14
and target heart rate zone, how to calculate, 14, 15
Henrickson, Debbie, 9
Hiking, planning vacation around, 88
Hinshaw, Jennifer, 9
Hogan, Ben, 117
Holyfield, Evander, 114

Ice skating, cooldown for, 267–68; and in-line skating compared, 215
Indirect calorimetry, defined, 251
Indoor exercise bikes. See Exercise bikes, indoor
Injuries
    cross training alternative during rehabilitation from, 86
    from ignoring pain, 262–63, 266
    from incorrect technique, 264
    lower body, deep water running for, 184
    and medical advice, 270–71
    from overuse, 86
    prevention through cross training, 3–4

from tennis, 86, 264
warm-ups to prevent,
267
In-line skating
exercise prescription for,
219
getting started in, 217
and ice-skating com-
pared, 215
illustrated, *19*
Potential Physical Fitness
Benefits Chart for, *216*
protective gear for, *216*
purchasing checklist for,
218–19
safety practices in, 281
In-Line Skating (Mark Powell and John Svensson),
217
Institute of Aerobic Re-
search, 209
International Swimming
Federation, 178
International Triathlon
Union, 155
Interval training, 21–22.
See also Anaerobic ex-
ercise
*Introduction to Nutrition,
Exercise and Health*
(Katch and McArdle),
259

Jackson, Bo, 2
Jenner, Bruce, 2
Jerome, John (*Staying
Supple: The Bountiful
Pleasures of Stretching*),
25
John Jay College, 91, 138,
174, 175, 176, 281

Cardiovascular Fitness
Center, 138, 175
Triathlon Club, 164
Johnson, Earvin "Magic,"
cross training program
of, 94–96, 108
Johnson, John. *See* Snead,
J. C., 118
Joel, Billy, 168
Jogging
as cross training activity
for swimming, 140
and running compared,
146–48
Jokl, Peter. *See* Mangi,
Richard, 261
Jordan, Michael, 1, 91
Joyner-Kersee, Jackie, 2,
279
Judo
aerobic activities as cross
training for, 121
cross training for, 120–22
philosophy of, 120–21
Potential Physical Fitness
Benefits chart for, *121*
quickness training for,
122
strength training for, 122
Jumping rope. *See* Rope
jumping

Karate
aerobic endurance exer-
cises for, 123
cross training for, 122–23
origins of, 122
Potential Physical Fitness
Benefits chart for, *123*
strength training for, 123
Kano, Jigaro, 120

developing upper body strength in, 74–75

major groups of skeletal, 42

manual resistance training with partner for toning of, 74

micro-tears in, as means of strengthening, 47

number of, in human body, 39, 42

smooth muscle, 42

straps for toning of, 62

strength training of, for racquet sports, 135–36

triceps stretch for golf flexibility, 118

tubing for toning of, 62

women's muscle tone, 45

Naismith, Dr. James, 106

National Organization of Mall Walkers, 145

National Sporting Goods Association, 223

Nenow, Mark, 9

Nettles, Craig, 105

New York City Marathon, 145

NordicSport Lateral Trainer, 191

Nordic Track Aerobic Cross-Trainer, 191

Oakley, Charles, 95

O'Brien, Dan, 2

Octopus Drill, for racquet sports, *134*

Orienteering

exercise prescription for, 246

getting started, 245–46

history of, in U.S., 244

Potential Physical Fitness Benefits chart for, *245*

O'Toole, Dr. Mary, 261

Oxygen consumption, defined, 252

Paddleball, Potential Physical Fitness Benefits chart for, *128*

Palance, Jack, 44

Physical fitness. *See also* Functional fitness; Potential Physical Fitness Benefits charts

achieving balance in, through cross training, 96–97

activities and sports ranked by potential benefits to, *289, 290*

and aerobic fitness, 4–5

Aerobic Point System program for, 250–51, 258

Assessment Form for, 77, 84

benefits of cross training for, 4

and body composition, 8

and cross-country ski machines, 86

and family fitness, 90

five components of, 4

and flexibility, 7–8

Flexibility Rating Scale for, 80

ful *Pleasures of Stretching* (John Jerome), 25
StairMaster, 202
Step classes. *See also* Aerobic dance
  described, 229–30
  Potential Physical Fitness Benefits chart for, *231*
  videotape for, *230*
Step machines
  advantages of, *203–4*
  as cross training activity for baseball, 99
  exercise prescription for, 205–6
  form for, 205
  Potential Physical Fitness Benefits chart for, *202;* for climbing machine (VersaClimber), *205*
  for tennis players, 86
  VersaClimber as variation of, 204
Strength training
  abdominal exercises for, 60–*61*
  for baseball, 100–101
  basic routine for, 48; positions in basic routine illustrated, *51–61*
  Bench Press Test for, 81, *82–83*
  benefits of, 5–6
  circuit training, 48
  cross-lateral transfer phenomenon in, 46
  duration of, discussed, 49
  four methods of, 46
  free weight for, 46
  frequency of, discussed, 49
  with gravitrons, 74–75

intensity of, 46
for judo, 122
for karate, 123
machines for, 46
manual resistance from partner for, 46
muscle exercise sequence for, 50
progression in, 47
for racquet sports, 135–36
sample workout for, 49–50
specificity in, 46
straps, bands, tubing for, 46
upper body, lower body alternation in, 49
weight-lifting for, 6
women discouraged from, 45
Stretching. *See also* Flexibility
  guidelines for, 26
  illustrated, *27–38*
  parts of body to be stretched, 62
Stroke sports. *See* Racquet sports
Svensson, John. *See* Powell, Mark, 217
Swimming. *See also* Triathlon
  as cross training activity for baseball, 99
  cross training for, 139–43
  cross training on terrain, when to, 139–40
  exercise prescription for beginners, 179–80
  50-Meter Sprint, 6-Week Training Program for, 141, *142*